NEUROCINEMA

NEUROCINEMA

WHEN FILM MEETS
NEUROLOGY

EELCO F. M. WIJDICKS

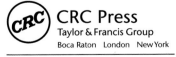

CRC Press
Taylor & Francis Group
Boca Raton   London   New York

CRC Press is an imprint of the
Taylor & Francis Group, an **informa** business

CRC Press
Taylor & Francis Group
6000 Broken Sound Parkway NW, Suite 300
Boca Raton, FL 33487-2742

Printed on acid-free paper
Version Date: 20140729

International Standard Book Number-13: 978-1-4822-4286-7 (Paperback)

Library of Congress Cataloging-in-Publication Data

Wijdicks, Eelco F. M., 1954- , author.
   Neurocinema : when film meets neurology / Eelco F.M. Wijdicks.
   p. ; cm.
   Includes bibliographical references and index.
   ISBN 978-1-4822-4286-7 (pbk. : alk. paper)
   I. Title.
   [DNLM: 1. Medicine in Art. 2. Motion Pictures as Topic. 3. Nervous System Diseases--psychology. 4. Neurology. 5. Physician's Role--psychology. 6. Physicians--psychology. WZ 331]

R702.5
777.896168--dc23   2014027940

Visit the Taylor & Francis Web site at
http://www.taylorandfrancis.com

and the CRC Press Web site at
http://www.crcpress.com

For Barbara, Coen, and Marilou

Contents

Preface

Coma, stroke, seizures, and spinal cord injury are conditions that appeal to screenwriters, and as we will find out, there are several feature films where neurologic disease unfurls as a plot element. Film directors know that neurologic disease impacts both mind and motility. Equally important, these films say as much about the consequences as they say about the disorder.

My central curiosity was to find out how these films are done. It should be interesting to deconstruct the neurologic representation in film. There are obvious questions to ask: How are neurologic disorders shown, and how accurately are they depicted? How is the practice of the neurologist represented? How do documentaries handle the seriousness of these disorders? Do films have educational value for neurology residents, and can the topic bring about a useful discussion?

This book is organized by the main neurologic conditions after selecting over 100 films. I divided the material into chapters that include discussions on neurologic disorders (Chapter 3), moral and ethical quandaries in major neurologic illnesses (Chapter 4), neurology as a subject of a documentary (Chapter 5), and what I call neurofollies (silly neurology), as frequently used in science fiction (Chapter 6).

Neurologic disorders in film are not so easy to find, and even titles such as *Coma*, *Brain*, *Dementia 13*, and *Vertigo* are about different themes. The films were found after using a variety of library and Internet resources, but the filmography mostly came from a personal file I have kept over the years. The selection criteria were broad and inclusive, but the films chosen had to have well-defined scenes showing the acting out of a neurologic disorder and its consequences. I also included documentary films, recognizing that documentaries are not free of bias. Sometimes they are what they are—overdramatizing and close to fiction.

Films that only tangentially mentioned neurologic signs and symptoms (e.g., "cause I get such a headache right through my skull—Bong Bong" [*Harry and Tonto*, 1974], spell from presumed toxin [*Safe*, 1997]) were not considered. Excluding these films was generally simple. TV series such as *Grey's Anatomy*, *House MD*, and *ER* have inserted neurologic disorders in their stories, and the nature of films and series made for TV is changing and now often closely approximating feature films. However, in order to maintain focus, films made for TV and TV series were also excluded, unless they involved a crucial topic that I felt was important. Finally, I have shied away from bottom feeder horror and slasher films because, I suppose, when it pertains to brains and gore, there is nothing we can learn here, and it is a dead end.

I recognize that this book inescapably remains a personal selection of films and topics, and it cannot be an exhaustive resource without the full availability of all distributed films (World cinema is thus underrepresented). All the films mentioned in this book should be available on DVD, YouTube, or media video stream sites (e.g., Netflix, Hulu, and Amazon).

The main premise of this book is to discuss a film (or two) that represents the salient aspects of a specific neurologic disorder and its impact. (*Spoiler alert*: Because many of these reviews have details about the films, they probably should be read after the film is seen.) These films should be seen fully and not just for one clip. Plots are summarized, key scenes are analyzed, some shots are parsed, and the discussions may illuminate what underlies the screenwriters' intentions. The selected film is then compared with other films that are worth watching, even if they contain only a single pertinent scene. To provide further context, each chapter has background information aimed mostly at physicians, but accessible for the nonmedical reader as well. The purpose of these essays is to elaborate on what is shown, but it is up to the reader/viewer to be fascinated, amused, or appalled by the film. Each chapter has text boxes containing dialogue lines that were chosen to draw the reader into the film and to highlight the themes. These conversational exchanges also accentuate the brilliant art of one-liner writing.

What more can be done with this information? I decided to judge these films but avoided a fail/pass decision, rating them instead on an ordinal scale. The traditional tools used by the neurologist are the reflex hammer (to test tendon and superficial reflexes) and a pin (to test sensation). The film's accuracy is thus qualified using a rating scale from one to four reflex hammers. Folly and absurdity are qualified using a rating scale from one to three pinpricks because these films are painful to watch. Rating a film with four reflex hammers required an unquestionably accurate neurologic representation. Rating a film with two or three reflex hammers required the presence of a teachable scene or some other interesting aspect. One reflex hammer indicated a serious misrepresentation. The pinpricks indicated—in a handful of unredeemable silly films—a representation that was really bad to even worse.

Screenwriters and directors may deviate from reality in order to produce a certain effect. Thus neurology may give way to the story, and such an approach may be permitted in the name of poetic license. At best it is just entertainment, and there may even be situations—walking out of the theater—where the physician (or neurologist) in the party may have to clarify what just happened. At worst, a departure from the truth may result in misperceptions by the general public. Some films are serious and comical at the same time, making it difficult to filter out problems with portrayal. This book, of course, has no formal film analysis and interpretation of its narrative structure because I lack the credentials to judge the artistry of filmmaking. I recognize the need for film directors to dramatize, the need to create a gripping and watchable film while skewing some of the reality, even after obtaining advice from medical professionals. I recognize that any art criticism is arbitrary and arguably pretentious. Some may say that such close scrutiny is not needed ("Hey, it's only a movie"), but gross misrepresentation of serious neurologic disease does no good to the lay public. The best filmmakers not only entertain, but also come face to face with the subject matter.

This may leave the reader wondering, where does the "neurocinema critic" come in? Neurologists might anticipate being troubled by the portrayal, but there are a considerable number of films that are accurate representations of acute or chronic neurologic disease. Neurologic disease can be devastating, and many of us will be stirred by the images placed before us within the context of some mordant dramas. I think many of these films are mandatory viewing, not only for specialists in the neurosciences, but for everyone else as well. Some documentaries are nearly impossible to watch, and some fiction films are comical, but all provide something to talk about.

For me, seeing a film is a fantastic experience. I am often asked, "Have you seen…?" or told, "You should see…!" and thus it is only natural to combine my profession with an interest of mine and to write about neurologic representation in film. I noticed early on that many films used acute neurology in their screenplays, and that fits my subspecialty. I wanted to put together a series of important fiction films and documentaries that I think few of the readers have seen or even heard about.

I hope the reader finds this collection of film critiques—summarized by the rubric *Neurocinema*—informative and educational, serious and amusing, and that it will lead to watching or rewatching these celebrated films.

It was a great pleasure to write about them.

Acknowledgments

Seeing neurology through film requires close observation and recognition of proper representations. This could only have been done with the help, criticism, and suggestions of colleagues with expertise other than mine. Many people have shared their knowledge with me. I would like to thank Joseph Duffy, Christopher Boes, Michael Silber, Eric Ahlskog, Bradley Boeve, Orhun Kantarci, Jerry Kaplan, Amulya NageswaraRao, Erik St. Louis, Anne Moessner, Ashley Sporer, and Jeffrey Ward. I thank Dr. Masashi Okubo for translating Japanese films and Dr. Girish Banwari for pointing out relevant films in Hindi cinema. Michel Toledano—neurologist and filmmaker—taught me much about Cinema with a capital C. Several filmmakers have been very helpful in providing material. I thank Scott Kirschenbaum, Richard Ledes, Vincent Straggas, and Banker White.

It is a nearly impossible struggle to obtain permission for the use of movie posters and stills. The following distributors, however, have kindly provided posters for the films discussed: Ferndale Films/Hell's Kitchen, Ltd.; El Deseo S.A.; Les Films du Losange; Music Box Films; and eOne Publicity. Permission has also been obtained from several other sources and is acknowledged in the figure captions. Portions of some vignettes have been published as reviews in *Neurology Today*. I thank Kay Ellis, *Neurology Today* editor, and Steven Goodrich, senior editor of *The Lancet Neurology*, both of whom have been very supportive and encouraging with each of these reviews.

I sincerely thank Lori Lynn Reinstrom for providing all the secretarial and editorial assistance these projects needed. She has been creative and even suggested films I should look into. I am especially grateful to the Section of Scientific Publications copy editors at Mayo Clinic for carefully reading the entire text (Alissa Baumgartner, John Hedlund, Angie Herron, and Ann Ihrke). I thank Jim Rownd for help in creating the beautiful cover and theater marquees. The production team (Amy Rodriguez) at CRC Press/Taylor & Francis has ably assisted me in improving the structure of the book and prose. I thank Lance Wobus, my editor at CRC Press/Taylor & Francis, for his encouragement and valuable commentary.

I dedicate this book to my wife and children—we see and talk movies all the time.

Neurofilm Collection

(Continued)

Neurologic Disorders *(Continued)*

Topic	Discussed Films
Cerebral palsy	*Gaby, A True Story, My Left Foot, Door to Door*
Autism spectrum disorders	*Fly Away, Adam, Rain Man, Extremely Loud & Incredibly Close*
Tourette's syndrome	*Niagara, Niagara, The Tic Code, Deuce Bigelow, Matchstick Men*
Dementia	*Iris, A Song for Martin, Away from Her, The Notebook, Memories of Tomorrow*
Parkinson's disease	*A Late Quartet, Love & Other Drugs*
Neurogenetics	*Lorenzo's Oil, The Cake Eaters, Extraordinary Measures, The Madness of King George*

Neuroethics

Topic	Discussed Films
Physician-assisted suicide	*You Don't Know Jack*
Self-determination	*Whose Life Is It Anyway? The Sea Inside, An Act of Murder, Million Dollar Baby*
Withdrawal of support from brain injury	*The Descendants, Steel Magnolias*
Family conflicts on care	*Critical Care*
Brain death and organ donation	*All About My Mother, 21 Grams*
Institutionalizing	*The Savages, Fred Won't Move Out*
Experimentation	*Extreme Measures*
Compassion fatigue	*The Death of Mr. Lazarescu*

Neurodocumentaries

Topic	Discussed Films
Alzheimer's disease	*You're Looking at Me Like I Live Here and I Don't, The Genius of Marian, The Forgetting, Extreme Love*
Huntington's disease	*Do You Really Want To Know?*
Multiple sclerosis	*When I Walk*
Motor neuron disease	*So Much So Fast, Living with Lew, I Am Breathing*
Aphasia after stroke	*After Words, Picturing Aphasia, Aphasia*
Poliomyelitis	*A Paralyzing Fear, Martha in Lattimore*
Traumatic brain injury	*The Crash Reel*
Rehabilitation	*Coma*

Neurofollies

Topic	Discussed Films
Enter the mind	*The Cell*
Psychic after coma	*The Dead Zone*
Total amnesia	*50 First Dates*
Enhancing brain function	*Limitless*
Intellectual disability to genius	*Charly*
Superintelligence	*Phenomenon*
Violent seizures	*The Terminal Man*
Computer-assisted neuronal activity	*Brain Waves*
Mind control	*Donovan's Brain*
Brain preservation	*The Brain That Wouldn't Die*

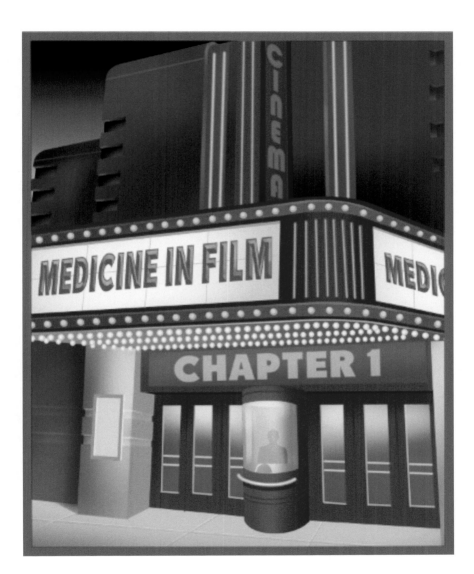

CHAPTER 1

Medicine in Film

You know the secret of being a good doctor, don't you?... You act like one.

The Good Doctor (2011)

In film and in reality, illness is often unexpected and accidental. Using serious illness as a plot device brings melodrama to the narrative arc. Filmmakers often perceive medicine as health interrupted by illness followed by disability or death, and this topic is an endless source of ideas and fictional inventions. Screenwriters have inserted life-threatening disorders—often suddenly diagnosed terminal cancer and more recently AIDS—into the story because they are unnerving to the audience and create tension in the narrative. Doctors often appear when the leading character in the film becomes sick, and over many years their portrayal has evolved from the general family doctor to medical specialists, parallel with subspecialization of medicine as a whole.

The medical specialties that screenwriters prefer the most are surgeons, psychiatrists, and pediatricians. Themes may be specific to the type of specialty, and of course, we have all seen the heroic lifesaving surgeon.

Filmmakers are very good at creating panicky epidemics. Dystopian viral outbreaks such as the avian flu have attracted filmmakers. Each of these films can be easily liable to the charge that it is nothing but scary mainstream movie entertainment. Medicine is also a topic of comedy, making fun of medical decisions and physicians. There is also a surplus of psychiatric disorders, mostly involving neuroses and addictions. There are numerous screwball comedies involving psychiatrists. Yet, in the end, medical diseases are rarely depicted in the major films (only three in Roger Ebert's book *The Great Movies,* comprising 300 reviews, and no entries in the magazine *Sight and Sound*'s Top 50 poll).

Medicine in film has been researched well, and the reader is referred to several texts, listed at the end of this chapter. For physicians, the representation of medicine—particularly in films of import—is always interesting, commonly fascinating, and sometimes laughable. Here we glimpse into the cinematic portrayal of hospitals, doctors, and diseases as a lead-in to the main topic of this book.

PORTRAYAL OF HOSPITALS

The depiction of medicine often starts outside the hospital and in ambulance runs (*Bringing Out the Dead* [1999]). Most of the time ambulances are presented as being in a state of chaos, with physicians questioning who is in charge. And of course we have the emergency department, where patients are rushed in with yelling and screaming staff and often a bloody mess. Because medical illness often involves trauma or a gunshot wound, we may get to see the operating room and the intensive care area. For dramatic purposes and to create further tension, a surgeon may be seen rushing out of the operating room to tell distressing news to family members (*Miami Vice* [2006]). In the recent film *Fruitvale Station* (2013), a surgeon enters the waiting room and tells an anxiously waiting family, "He did not make it."

Intensive care units (ICUs) or surgical trauma units usually show the actor after polytrauma—packed in and in traction. Most remarkable is that sometimes the sound of the patient's heartbeat is heard—as it is in the operating room—becoming fast when the patient is in distress. (Note that ICUs do have alarms, but no audible heartbeat can be heard from the equipment used.) The ventilator shown in the ICU often looks similar to the one used in the operating room (bellows included).

Medical institutions are not always depicted accurately. Veterans Affairs (VA) hospitals are commonly shown, usually in the war-film genre. VA hospitals are either appalling places (*Coming Home* [1978], *Born on the Fourth of July* [1989]) or places where bureaucracy leads to nothing but frustration (*Article 99* [1992]).

The most shocking institution is the psychiatric hospital. In 1975, the movie *One Flew over the Cuckoo's Nest* cemented a dramatic negative depiction of the psychiatrist and psychiatric nursing staff, and

Shutter Island (2003) was a film noir, with the criminally insane in shackles. Hospital drama continues to interest filmmakers, and atrocious treatment predominates.

PORTRAYAL OF PHYSICIANS

Films released in the 1930s and 1940s showed physicians as fine country doctors who were simple and compassionate, inserting their lives into the tragedies of patients. Over time, the portrayal dramatically changed, with film also introducing major medical ethical issues such as mercy killing and abortion.

Many directors have used physicians in film—most of them male, attractive, and witty, although the sympathetic portrayal of the character varies depending on the needs of the script. When the doctor enters the scene, he is usually meticulously dressed in a crisp white coat.

In the United States, the *Doctor Kildare* TV and movie series became a classic in the depiction of physicians, nurses, and administrators, showing a virtually perfect world of medicine. The series included *Dr. Kildare's Crisis* (1940) and *Dr. Kildare's Wedding Day* (1941) with the classic line of dialogue, "Doctors doctor for 24 hours a day. The rest of the time he can't be a husband." A world where physicians could not combine their profession with marriage was portrayed, and full commitment to the profession was necessary. There were very few female doctors in early feature films (e.g., *The Girl in White* [1952]). Female doctors appear in numerous later films, often to show some gentle flirtation or even marriage (Erika Marozsan in *Feast of Love* [2007]).

There were many other problematic portrayals of the medical profession. One of the most notorious is *The Interns* (1962), where a group of young doctors is moving into practice. The nursing staff is told, "Never talk to the interns. They are all sex maniacs."

The portrayal of doctors has evolved from the dedicated solo general practitioner to a character study of the arrogant, intimidating hotshot surgeon. In *Doc Hollywood* (1991), Michael J. Fox stated, "Beverly Hills, plastic surgery, the most beautiful women in the world. What do these three things have in common? Answer: Me in one week."

Gynecologists occasionally appear, even as the main actor in one movie—Richard Gere in Robert Altman's *Dr. T and the Women* (2000). Gynecologists are also involved with birth traumas. *Rosemary's Baby* (1968) is the major representation of hysterical pregnancy, rape fantasies, and other absurdities such as germinating a devil child. All of this has one theme, which is to shock and create a troubling feeling for the moviegoer.

Because there are many films portraying people with psychiatric disorders, the portrayal of psychiatrists has been well analyzed. They have been categorized as competent and caring (Dr. Bergen, played by Judd Hirsch in *Ordinary People* [1980]), neurotic and comical (Richard Dreyfuss as Dr. Marvin in *What About Bob?* [1991]), and evil experimenters (Dr. Hannibal Lecter, played by Anthony Hopkins in *Silence of the Lambs* [1991]).

The social and professional status of physicians is high, and their offices are typically shown as being large, with large cluttered desks. There are quite a few surgeons who drive sports cars and live in lush country homes. Some films discuss the salaries of specialists, most notably in *Crisis* (1950), where the neurosurgeon (played by Cary Grant) says "My fee? I usually charge 10% of the patient's income." In *Drunken Angel* (1948), the physician says to his patient, "I warn you, my fees are very high—I always overcharge people who eat and drink too much." But there are more peculiarities. Some films emphasize addictions by physicians, or physicians practicing while intoxicated, such as the general surgeon (Alec Baldwin) in *Malice* (1993) and the heart surgeon (Kirk Harris) stealing drugs from the hospital to trade for cocaine in *Intoxicating* (2003).

Screenwriters have toiled carefully over portrayals of specialists, and a summary of their specialty characterizations is shown in Table 1.1.

Nurses in film were in a role of servitude for many decades. Often in the nurse–physician relationship, the nurse played a lesser role and endured harassment and verbal abuse. Nurses were typically in awe of the doctors, because "they always know best." Doctors were also seen as major marriage material and incited jealousy among the nurses.

The relationship of physicians and nursing staff is also often confrontational. In *Critical Care* (1979), there is an important dialogue where the nurse questions whether the care of a patient in a persistent vegetative state needs continuation. The physician answers, "It's important that we say that we did everything," to which the nurse replies, "That's doctor-speak for 'we put this patient through hell before he died.'"

Exploitive relationships are common in the movies, and loss of physician boundaries is sometimes used as a plot device. In virtually every film involving doctors, there is a barrier between patient and doctor—only to

TABLE 1.1   Characterization of Medical Specialties in Film

Anesthesia	"Anesthesia is the easiest thing in the world until something goes wrong. It's 99 percent boredom and 1 percent scared-shitless panic." (*Coma* [1978])
Surgery	"A surgeon's job is to cut—get in, fix it, and get out." (*The Doctor* [1991])
	"You do not think much of surgeons. Not as much as they think of themselves." (*The Interns* [1962])
Intensive care	"Jesus brought Lazarus back from the dead, but he did it only once. People were amazed we did it every day." (*Critical Care* [1997])
Family medicine	"I am just a small-town doctor who pushes aspirin to the elderly." (*Eve's Bayou* [1997])
Dermatology	"The patient never gets better and never gets sick." (*Young Dr. Kildare* [1938])
Neurology	"Those damn neurologists, they think they can run the world." (*EDtv* [1999])
Neurosurgery	"It is like Russian roulette. In one hand you have a revolver called treatment and the other side a revolver called no treatment." (*The English Surgeon* [2007])
Psychiatry	"Evaluate, medicate, vacate." (*12 Monkeys* [1995])

be broken later—or the physician seeks a relationship with a family member (Diane Keaton in *Something's Gotta Give* [2003] and Keri Russell in *Waitress* [2007]). *Critical Care* (Chapter 4) is also one of many examples of movies in which doctors go overboard. This time, the daughter of a patient develops a sexual relationship with the attending physician ("You are the first doctor I've met who seems human").

Medical biographic films (biopics) have rarely been made, and most of these have involved researchers, such as *The Story of Louis Pasteur* (1936) (vaccinations), *Dr. Ehrlich's Magic Bullet* (1940) (ether discovery), *The White Angel* (1936) (heroic nurses, in this case Florence Nightingale), and *Sister Kenny* (1946) (treatment of poliomyelitis; see Chapter 3). There are some more recent biopics, but they involve the psychiatry greats Freud and Jung in *A Dangerous Method* (2011) and the sexual researcher Alfred Kinsey in *Kinsey* (2004).

PORTRAYAL OF DISEASES

Cinematic diseases run a similar course to reality, but the mortality rates are higher (*Love Story* [1970], *Terms of Endearment* [1983]). Cardiopulmonary resuscitation has been shown in a number of films (*Bringing Out the Dead* [1999]) and as expected the intervention has spectacularly good outcomes, even after the physician has pronounced the patient dead (*The Girl in White* [1950]).

Cinema has dealt with diseases in multifarious ways, but rarely have such films become classics. Kurosawa's *Ikiru* (1952) deals with a man with inoperable gastric cancer and is an example of a film that addresses disease as its main theme. A full discussion of major medical diseases is outside the scope of this book, but Table 1.2 shows some of the more recognizable films. Doctors may also get sick (*The Doctor* [1991]), and directors often shape this into a life-changing event, which it often is.

Directors often find their topics for a screenplay where medicine interfaces with other disciplines, such as ethics and psychology. There has been substantial analysis of film by bioethicists, psychologists, and sociologists, and many themes can be detected. For instance, there are multiple explanations for Dr. Isak Borg's character in Ingmar Bergman's *Wild Strawberries* (1960). The themes of pity and regret, guilt, family dysfunctionality, religious doubt, fear of failing exams, and fear of death have all been considered by film critics. Dr. Borg is an emeritus professor of bacteriology, soon to be awarded

TABLE 1.2   Characterization of Medical Diseases in Film

Disorder	Film Examples
Cancer	*Ikiru* (1952)
	Cries and Whispers (1972)
	The Barbarian Invasions (2003)
HIV	*Philadelphia* (1993)
	Dallas Buyers Club (2013)
Alcoholism	*Leaving Las Vegas* (1995)
	Crazy Heart (2009)
Viral epidemic	*Outbreak* (1995)
	Contagion (2011)
Myocardial infarction	*Something's Gotta Give* (2003)
Neurofibromatosis/Proteus syndrome	*Elephant Man* (1980)
	Under the Skin (2013)
Bipolar disorder, schizophrenia	*Mr. Jones* (1993)
	A Beautiful Mind (2001)

Jubeldoctor [50-year anniversary of doctoral thesis], and he reminisces about his life. Because Bergman had such a good understanding of psychoanalysis, one could argue that psychologists and psychiatrists should watch and analyze his movies—and perhaps nothing else.

CONCLUSION

Medicine in film can be approached and studied from many angles. We can break it up as depictions of disorders, specialists, medical institutions, and medical biographies. Many films are provocative (often involving psychiatric depictions), doctors are not always the good supporters of patients, and there is a good dose of grandiosity in surgeons. Physicians with a one-track mind who are not fazed by alternative explanations are a common theme. The bedside manner is ridiculed often by depicting patronizing and domineering behavior, but there are examples of kindness and compassion, too. The audience may cynically say that such characterizations are no different from the world we are living in.

Most screenwriters are not physicians, and they usually do not adapt a screenplay from a book written by a physician. Exceptions are the Scottish writer A.J. Cronin, whose books spanned a number of films in Indian cinema, and of course, Michael Crichton and Oliver Sacks. Films may in some way reflect how screenwriters and directors see physicians, and it is not a pretty picture. The next chapter shows us how neurologists fare.

Further Reading

Alexander M, Pavlov A, Lenahan P. *Cinemeducation: A comprehensive guide to using film in medical education.* London: Radcliffe Publishing, 2005.

Colt H, Quadrelli S, Friedman L. *The picture of health: Medical ethics and the movies.* New York: Oxford University Press USA, 2011.

Dans PE. *Doctors in the movies: Boil the water and just say aah.* Lansing, MI: Medi-Ed Press, 2000.

Gabbard K, Gabbard GO. *Psychiatry and the cinema.* Chicago: University of Chicago Press, 1987.

Glasser B. *Medicinema: Doctors in film.* London: Radcliffe Publishing, 2010.

Harper G, Moor A. *Signs of life: Medicine in cinema.* London: Wallflower Press, 2005.

Robinson DJ. *Reel psychiatry: Movie portrayals of psychiatric conditions.* Port Huron, MI: Rapid Psychler Press, 2003.

Shapshay S. *Bioethics at the movies.* Baltimore: Johns Hopkins University Press, 2009.

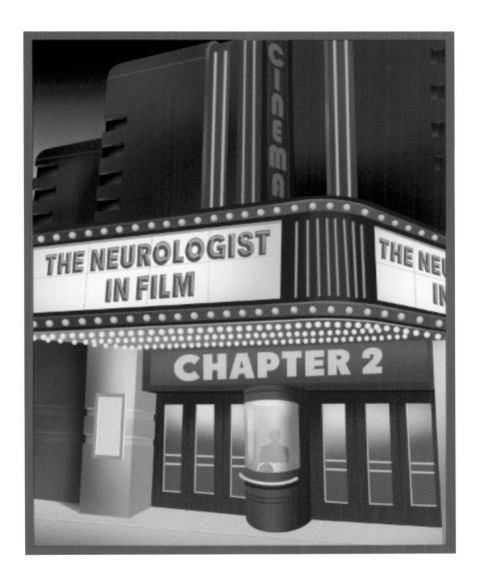

CHAPTER 2

The Neurologist in Film

Well, we called for a neurologist a half hour ago.

State of Play (2009)

What did the neurologist say?… He does not know.

Regarding Henry (1991)

Medicine is specialized, and expertise is divided over multiple areas. Physicians have a good idea what these fields entail. For everyone else, the question is: What is a neurologist? The American Academy of Neurology (AAN) defines a neurologist as "a medical doctor with specialized training in diagnosing, treating and managing disorders of the brain and nervous system." According to the AAN website, the disorders that neurologists treat are Alzheimer's disease and other dementias, brain injury and concussion, brain tumors, epilepsy, migraine and other headaches, multiple sclerosis, myasthenia gravis, peripheral neuropathy, amyotrophic lateral sclerosis, Parkinson's disease and other movement disorders, sleep disorders, spinal cord injury, and stroke. Many neurologists have been trained in a subspecialty, and acute disorders are often seen by neurointensivists, vascular neurologists, and epileptologists.

We do not know how much information screenwriters have available when neurologic disorders are considered. Similarly, moviegoers—when they see neurologists and neurologic disease on the screen—may be largely incognizant of this part of medicine.

So let us start with neurologists and see how they come across in cinema. Not surprisingly, neurologists were previously usually shown in a subsidiary role, not as protagonists. It may be that little is known of neurologists, and partly because this specialty is comparatively young. The same may apply to neurosurgeons—a specialty that came even later. It could also be because neurologic diagnoses and examinations do not move a narrative forward. It could also be the result of "neurophobia"— neurology is just too mysterious (an attitude shared by some medical students). Or it could simply be because screenwriters prefer surgeons, psychiatrists, and family doctors, or they may just keep the specialty of the doctor unknown.

Oddly enough, when the canon of films involving medical issues is examined, there are quite a few cinematic depictions of neurologists— but it is not a pretty picture. When neurologists appear on the screen, they usually run the full spectrum of caricatures and clichés. So before immersing ourselves in the discussion of cinematic depictions of a wide variety of neurologic disorders, it would be good to look at the cinematic traits of the neurologist. As we will see, neurologists are generally not depicted as go-getters; rather, they seem to move quite slowly and deliberately.

A FOUNDER OF NEUROLOGY IN FILM

Clinical neurology knows many founders. In the United Kingdom, Thomas Willis (1621–1675) coined the term *neurology* in his book *Cerebri Anatome*, followed by John Hughlings Jackson (1835–1911), who added many ideas to what would become a neurologic approach. In the United States, the development of the field came later and was modeled after French and British neurology, with the first role models being William Hammond (1828–1900), who wrote the first American textbook of neurology, *A Treatise on Diseases of the Nervous System*, and Silas Weir Mitchell (1829–1914). Many American neurologists also briefly trained in London at the National Hospital for the Paralysed and Epileptic in Queen Square.

Neurologists often had a psychiatry practice, and because of this link with psychiatry and particularly with hysteria, this caught the attention of at least one filmmaker. One feature film, *Augustine* (2012), directed by Alice Winocour, is devoted fully to a neurologist who was arguably the most influential of all—Dr. Jean-Martin Charcot (1825–1893), chair of Clinique des Maladies du Système Nerveux at La Salpêtrière (Figure 2.1).

He was widely consulted, and his ideas were universally accepted and never questioned—at least not in France at the time.

Although Charcot's contributions to neurology are legendary (two eponyms, description of amyotrophic lateral sclerosis and multiple sclerosis), his studies of female hysteria cemented his international fame. For Charcot, the neurologist, *hystérie* was a *névrose functionelle* and not psychiatry, and for a long time he was convinced there was a structural basis for the symptoms. Charcot was well known for his well-attended

(a)

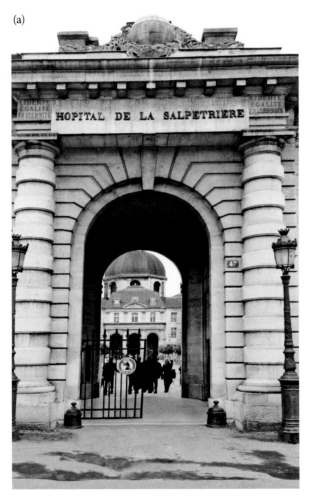

FIGURE 2.1 (a) Entrance of l'hôpital de la Salpêtrière in Paris.

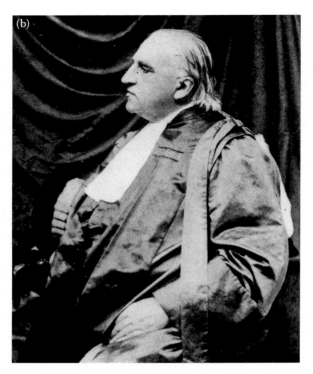

FIGURE 2.1 (*Continued*)   (b) Jean-Martin Charcot.

clinical demonstrations showing the effects of touching—usually by his assistants—of certain skin areas that could induce an hysterical attack. Charcot's treatment of young afflicted women (and also men) included hypnosis and, most memorably, the *compresseur ovarien* (an abdominal vice with a knob applying pressure to the ovary); and both could stop the spells. Charcot, his school, and the hysterical attacks have been described in numerous books, but most writers have taken significant artistic license.

In *Augustine*, Charcot is played by the great actor Vincent Lindon and is surrounded by admiring neurologists, further increasing his standing. The neurologist Bourneville (who discovered the disorder tuberous sclerosis) is in here, but he has no significant dialogue. Charcot and his patient Augustine are the main focus of the film. The manifestations of *la grande hystérie* are played by Soko (French actress Stéphanie Sokolinski), and we get quite a show. There is loud applause by all the attending neurologists after each hysterical attack. The movie shows hypnosis with a tuning fork and the patient following a small mirror that results in a spell (Figure 2.2).

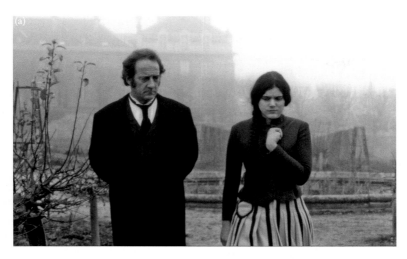

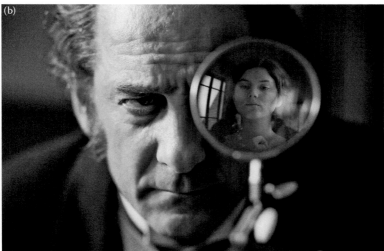

FIGURE 2.2 (a) Vincent Lindon as Charcot and Soko as Augustine in *Augustine*. Note the functional arm posture. (b) Charcot trying to hypnotize Augustine. (Photos provided by courtesy of Music Box Films: Charcot © Dharamsala Photo. J.C. Lother Charcot and Augustine: © Dharamsala Photo.)

The hysterical attacks are well done and very real, with a typical *arc en cercle* (arching body backwards).

Augustine also shows important aspects of the neurologic examination in a patient with so-called functional (not explained by disease) symptoms and is of interest because examination of the "functional" patient is quite common for neurologists. It shows the exact symmetric loss of sensation (dramatically indicated in this film with a big red pencil by Charcot), patches of hypo- and hypersensitivity, loss of smell in one nostril only, different types of color blindness in each eye, and a forcefully closed eye due to unilateral blepharospasm, called here "the hysterical wink." Augustine also displays a hysterical contracture.

The movie also suggests that Charcot was sexually attracted to Augustine and that this attraction at some point would overwhelm him. *Augustine* is based on a real patient of Charcot, but that is where the comparison ends, and the film becomes nothing but a psycho-erotic thriller. The film may be a distorted, overblown view on a chauvinist doctor's behavior. La Salpêtrière was a public women's hospital, and the physicians were all male, but even if Charcot's behavior was authoritarian, one cannot conclude misogyny. (A similar suggestion of erotic transference was made in John Huston's film *Freud* [1962], where Sigmund Freud massages the back of the completely undressed patient Dora—one of his famous case histories.)

Augustine is a must-see for neurologists. After all, how often do we get to see one of the pioneers of neurology on-screen? It is possible that in future period films, the neurologist's link to psychiatry could potentially typecast these early giants in the field.

MODERN NEUROLOGISTS IN FILM

Portrayals have included the aloof neuroscientist studying a rare neurologic disease (Bill Murray in *The Royal Tenenbaums* [2001]), the discompassionate curmudgeon (Patrick Chesnais in *The Diving Bell and the Butterfly* [2007]), and the glib unethical researcher (Gene Hackman in *Extreme Measures* [1996]).

The neurologist Oliver Sacks served as a model in two major feature films. In *Awakenings* (1990), Oliver Sacks is Dr. Sayer, played by Robin Williams. His character is the bearded, spectacled, coy neurologist discovering a cure for encephalitis lethargica. (According to Oliver Sacks—and after Robin Williams spent some time with him—the actor started to look like his identical twin brother with the same mannerisms.) In *The Royal Tenenbaums*, the much nerdier Raleigh St. Clair (played by Bill Murray) is not only modeled after Oliver Sacks, but a parody of his work (which usually contains highly unusual neurologic cases) is also featured. In *The Royal Tenenbaums*, Dr. St. Clair writes a book entitled *The Peculiar*

Neurodegenerative Inhabitants of the Kazawa Atoll and is seen studying a rare disorder of amnesia, dyslexia, and color blindness combined with a highly acute sense of hearing—a preposterous combination of clinical signs.

Apart from these Sacks-like satires, in most other films, the neurologist is like any physician, but sympathetic depictions are few and far between. After reviewing many films, I found there is enough information to discuss the portrayal of communication skills, diagnostic competence, and even the neurologic examination. Here are some tidbits to illustrate that.

First, how does the neurologist relay information? In *Declaration of War* (2011), the parents of a child afflicted with a brainstem tumor are approached by a pediatric neurologist who, to say the least, is not overflowing with compassion. She barges into the room with her entourage, looks at the child, tells the parents the child needs a CT scan, leaves, and has an assistant explain the details. Later, her inexplicable medical jargon and pompous attitude totally confuse the distraught parents.

The neurologist in *Good Bye, Lenin!* (2003) explains coma after resuscitation and leaves the family with the uncertainty of the patient ever awakening again. When the patient awakens after being comatose for eight months, they are again told that outcome still may be problematic.

The neurologist in *Iris* (2001), after Iris completes a word-naming test, tells her that her dementia is implacable. After Iris asks what he means, he says it's inexorable. She tells him that it won't win, and he counters, "It will win."

The neurologist in *A Song for Martin* (2001) suggests to the patient with Alzheimer's and his spouse that it is best not to use medication but to use mental gymnastics and love.

In the film *Go Now* (1995), the neurologist of a patient with suspected multiple sclerosis shuffles papers while eating a sandwich and cannot find test results. He says, "No results here…bit of a cock up." He then suggests that the patient return to the office in a month stating, "I am on holiday."

In *Garden State* (2004), the neurologist Dr. Cohen sees the protagonist for brief, intense, split-second headaches. (The scene shows a room filled with diplomas and achievements extending to the ceiling.) "Mr. Andrew Largeman, there is absolutely nothing wrong with you…just kidding… How would I know that? What can I do for you today?"

From these depictions of communication with families we can only conclude that the neurologist is often authoritarian, aloof, unrealistic, or without compassion.

However, there is some good out there, too. In *The Dreamlife of Angels* (1998), the neurologist played by Jean-Michel Lemayeux explains coma quite well to a visiting friend. "She is unconscious, she can't communicate. She can't talk or move. She won't answer you. We are watching for any sign of her waking or of an improvement." He asks the friend to watch for changes in her condition, and he provides compassionate support.

A more recent neurologist, in *The Descendants* (2012), discusses catastrophic brain injury well. "She will never be the way she was, Matt. We know that now. She may last several days to weeks".

Second, how is the competence of the neurologist portrayed? The neurologist's competency is questioned by the patient or the family in some films (*Go Now* [1995] and *Memories of Tomorrow* [2006]), most notably in the film *A Late Quartet* (2012), where the neurologist suggests a diagnosis of Parkinson's disease on the basis of a few simple tests. In *Memories of Tomorrow* (2007), the neurologist is young and seemingly inexperienced. When the neurologist tells the patient (Ken Watanabe) he has early Alzheimer's disease, the patient asks him how many years he has been practicing and laughs out loud at the neurologist when he hears it is only 10 years. The neurologist in this film is all business, prim and proper, and in a neat uncluttered office. After the second visit, the patient is told the positron emission tomography (PET) scan is diagnostic for Alzheimer's disease. The patient runs out of the office to a ledge on the roof of the hospital to commit suicide. The neurologist convinces him not to jump and to "have hope."

In *The Savages* (2007), Mr. Savage (Philip Bosco), disoriented and agitated, is restrained in the hospital, while his children, Jon and Wendy (played by Laura Linney and the late Philip Seymour Hoffman) are deciding how to put him in a nursing home. The neurologist calls his condition vascular dementia, but because he sees no stroke (CT scan is shown), he believes that with his disinhibition, aggression, and masked facies and blank stare, it is more likely Parkinson's disease. When the children ask him what to expect, he tells them he will likely die from cardiac complications. Soon they are seen reading books on the basics of dementia and Parkinson's disease and the real diagnosis is never revealed to the flustered children.

In *Lorenzo's Oil* (1991), the young boy Lorenzo is seen by a pediatric neurologist who finds nothing wrong. "The EEG is normal, skull x-ray is normal, CT is normal. I do not know what to tell you. This boy is neurologically intact." When the parents suggest some parasitic infection, the neurologist looks surprised and skeptical. Another pediatric neurologist suggests that "it could be any one of a dozen things," and admits him for tests. (The scene shows a hearing test with tuning fork, pupil reflex, electroencephalography [EEG], and CT scan, all with a dramatic opera soundtrack.) Finally, the diagnosis is revealed by Professor Nikolais—played by Peter Ustinov with bow tie and all—sitting behind a grand desk in a grand office.

These examples illustrate that when the cinematic depiction of the neurologist's competency is concerned, there is a constant uncertainty about the diagnosis and rarely transparency for family members. Neurologists sound rather vague and discombobulated.

How is the neurologic examination portrayed in film? The neurologic examination shown is fragmented, out of order, and bizarre. This is to be expected. As moviegoers know, a physical examination in film often consists of a doctor arriving with a large bag, listening to the patient, and stating with great certainty what is wrong or, equally often, that no one has to be concerned. However, this is different with the neurologic examination, which has always been elusive for nonneurologists and thus screenwriters. Not so much the tendon reflexes—reflex hammers are ubiquitously used by doctors in film—but it is the abnormal mental examination that has filmmakers thinking, and most of what we see in film is strange. It appears that some elements of the examination have been used by directors, without a full understanding of what these elements test and what they mean. Physicians and neurologists will be amused. A few examples follow. In *Crisis* (1950), Cary Grant plays Dr. Ferguson, a neurosurgeon (Chapter 3). He asks his patient to stretch out his arms, and his left arm (holding a cigarette) starts to drift downward followed by a loud cry, cramp, head turn, and unconsciousness for several seconds. He then performs a funduscopic examination ("There is great pressure.") and finds a visual-field defect.

In *Reversal of Fortune* (2005), Sunny von Bülow (played by Glenn Close) is found in a diabetic coma and is examined by a nervous neurologist in the emergency department who calls for an EEG (and not a CT scan) after performing a funduscopy.

In *The Men* (1950), a sensory examination is shown. Marlon Brando, as Bud, is a paraplegic who is tested by Dr. Brock. A safety pin is touched to the skin with the dull and sharp sides, and the doctor even simulates a touch without actually touching the skin in an effort to determine if the patient is guessing.

The most interesting depiction of a full neurologic examination (and neurologist behavior in an acute setting) is in *The Death of Mr. Lazarescu* (2005). The examination, however, is a bit all over the place. The film is about Mr. Lazarescu (Chapter 4), who has been complaining of headache and abdominal pain the entire day but is not cared for. After being sent out of a crowded emergency room, he arrives in another hospital, and one of the staff notes an asymmetry in his response. She calls the neurologist—Dr. Dragos Popescu (played by Adrian Titieni). When he enters the emergency room, he does not introduce himself and asks for the patient's name. He sits down at the bedside and immediately has him repeat an impossibly complex phrase ("Thirty-three storks on the roof of Mr. Kogalniceaunu."). He then follows with testing of forehead sensation followed by testing of eye tracking, testing of pupil reflexes to light, finger-to-nose testing (it shows the patient misses on the right), testing of finger strength by asking to squeeze, testing for drift (there is a mild drift on the right), testing leg strength by having him bend his knees (he has a subtle weakness), and asking him to walk. The medic warns him that he cannot walk, but the doctor ignores her completely, and the patient nearly falls to the ground. The doctor then proceeds with tendon reflexes (he taps with a reflex hammer on the muscle rather than the tendon). Then he goes back to testing of speech and shows him his wristwatch and asks him what it is. With a wrong answer, he concludes there is a subdural hematoma, and he tells the nurse, whom he flirts with (rubbing her shoulders and calling her *mi amor*), that it is urgent. He tells the patient he has a blood clot on the brain but also not to worry because the operation is simple and like surgery for appendicitis. Surely for neurologists, this depiction of a neurologic examination is not only taking a few liberties but is outright farcical.

CONCLUSION

Reviewing these films is a stark reminder that there is a stereotype of a neurologist who appears as the intellectual, aloof neuroscientist and head-scratcher (bow tie included)—not much different from his counterpart, the psychiatrist. This is understandable because both specialties have similar roots. The character study of one of the founders of neurology, Jean-Martin Charcot, is very much worth watching as a period piece and for parts of the neurologic examination of the patient with imagined neurologic illness, but of course the story is wrong.

In films depicting the modern neurologist, the scenes—when seen together—may even illustrate another motif. Diagnostic skills are way off, and often there is uncertainty about what is going on. In several films, the neurologist is denigrating.

Do these films help us to understand the neurologist any better? Of course they do not. In film, it is hard to feel a kinship toward them, and almost never does a fiction film provide a useful insight into our current practice. Nonmedical viewers will continue to ask what a neurologist really "does." We, as neurologists, will have to wait for a better depiction of our field with its many subspecialties and its many disorders that require timely recognition and complex management, even if there is no curative treatment. These disorders and their portrayal in cinema—right or wrong—are the focus of the next few chapters.

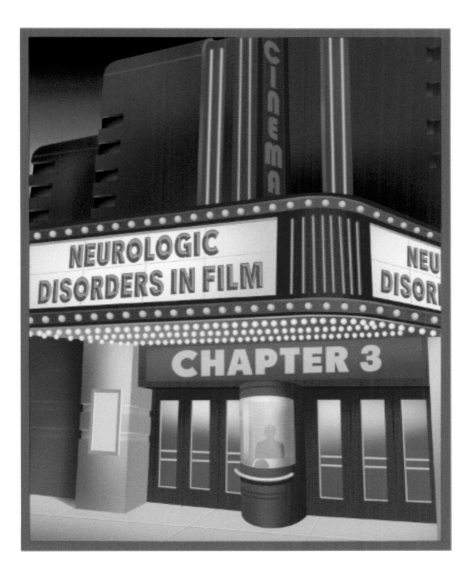

CHAPTER 3

Neurologic Disorders in Film

There is no point in going on living. That is how it is. I know it can only get worse. Why would I inflict this on us, on you and me?

Amour (2012)

INTRODUCING MAIN THEMES

The next three chapters are the core of the book, and we start with reviewing the major fiction films that portray neurologic disease.

When specifically asked, physicians—and certainly neurologists—will likely think that the portrayal in film of neurologic disorders is inaccurate, perhaps even absurd. By its very nature, theatrical portrayal is always in some way contrived, and embellishment of a new neurologic handicap might be expected in the art form we are discussing here. Indeed, there is some exaggeration, but this chapter will show that the portrayal of the major syndromes and clinical signs can approach reality quite closely, and it often is deeply affecting. Many films (i.e., directors and screenwriters) have earned their renown for a good reason.

So how do actors render neurologic disease? What is the impact neurologic disease has on relationships, work, even creativity? How does the drama before us articulate the seriousness and the vicissitudes of some neurologic disorders?

The main themes in *Neurocinema* are sudden confrontation with a major neurologic illness, disability from chronic neurologic disease, and inability to lead a normal life anymore. Acute neurologic conditions produce sudden plot twists and are thus frequently used in screenplays. Some filmmakers use a variety of cinematic techniques to show confusion (having the camera turning 360 degrees around a person), seizures (loud shrieking sounds), and visual disturbances (zooming in and out and blurring of the camera lens), but none approaches the personal experience of being struck by a neurologic disorder.

Neurologic disease can be seen in three scenarios. The first and most visible one is a film based on or inspired by a true story. These films come naturally because the story is often well researched and has originated from a personal memoir. Examples are *Reversal of Fortune*, *The Sea Inside*, *Lorenzo's Oil*, *My Left Foot*, *Iris*, and more recently, *The Intouchables*. All these films have distinct qualities, and the neurologic disorder is a vital thread, but it still needs a great actor to do it right. Beyond those examples are several more underappreciated and less frequently seen films that are chiefly concerned with one specific topic that drives the plot, for example, *A Late Quartet*, *Side Effects*, and *The Tic Code*.

Finally, there is a category where neurology is fleetingly mentioned in one or two scenes, maybe briefly as part of the story, but not as part of the main plot. Some have notable moments, and examples of films in this category include *Steel Magnolias*, *The Dreamlife of Angels*, *The Lookout*, *Barbara*, and *Drugstore Cowboy*. No explanation is necessary in comedies, but they are mentioned here if they address a very strange depiction. (The real follies are presented in Chapter 6.) Hopefully, each of these essays offers enough grist for further discussion.

COMA IN FILM

Reversal of Fortune (1990); starring Jeremy Irons, Glenn Close, and Ron Silver; directed by Barbet Schroeder, written by Nicholas Kazan; Golden Globe for best actor (Jeremy Irons); distributed by Warner Brothers.

Rating

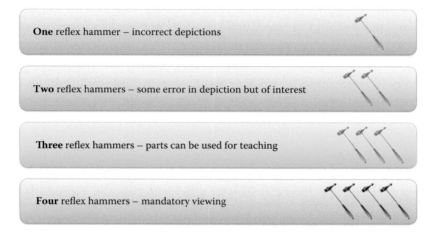

Talk to Her (Hable con Ella) (2002); starring Javier Cámara, Darío Grandinetti, Leonor Watling, Geraldine Chaplin, and Rosario Flores; written and directed by Pedro Almodóvar; Academy Award for best original screenplay, Golden Globe Award for best foreign language film, and BAFTA Award for best film not in English language and for best original screenplay; distributed by Sony Pictures.

Rating

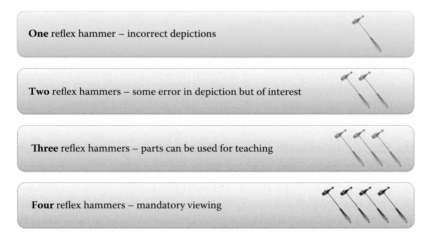

Criticism and Context

These films are about coma, most simply defined as a state in which the patient is unaware of his surroundings, does not awaken in response to a strong stimulus or pinch, and does not speak or open eyes. When the arms move, the responses are withdrawal or reflexive and not purposeful. The use of coma and prolonged coma (persistent vegetative state) in the movies seems ubiquitous, but there is still a comparatively small number in feature films.

Reversal of Fortune is the true story of Sunny and Claus von Bülow, her "comas," and how her condition and Claus' murder charge played out in the courts. Sunny von Bülow (Glenn Close) has several bouts of diabetic coma, and she does not awaken from the third one. She is found lying in the bathroom with her husband (Jeremy Irons) acting uninterested because he expects her to wake up (she did it twice before). "Please call an ambulance," is spoken matter-of-factly, without any sense of urgency. Sunny ends up in the emergency room and is examined (Chapter 2), but she remains in a vegetative state. She is shown lying immobile with eyes closed, a tracheostomy, and accurate positioning of her arms and wrists to mimic contractures. For dramatic effect, the mise-en-scène is a single hospital bed set in dazzling blue, adding to the loneliness and devastation. In real life, Sunny von Bülow died nearly 28 years later, remaining all the while in a persistent vegetative state attended by private nurses on the Upper East Side of New York.

Quotable Lines of Dialogue

Reversal of Fortune

Sunny von Bülow

I never woke from this coma, and I never will—I am in what doctors call a persistent vegetative state—a vegetable. According to medical experts, I could stay like this for a very long time—brain dead—body better than ever.

The film shows each of these hypoglycemic comas well. (Glenn Close narrates and recounts each of these comas—"first coma," "second coma.") There is even a mention of bradycardia and hypothermia, so common in these types of comas. Claus von Bülow instructs the maid to "get something warm, a blanket or anything you can find." However, she would not awaken despite superb medical care ("all this activity was pointless"). The sensational trial—guilty twice, acquitted eventually—of Claus von Bülow (Jeremy Irons) is the major part of the movie. There is an implication in the film that earlier episodes of diabetic hypoglycemic coma in Sunny von Bülow involved the use of needles containing barbiturates and valium as well as insulin. This film presents a very accurate portrayal of diabetic coma, and edited clips can be used for teaching. This is an uncomfortable reality when there is long-lasting hypoglycemia and the patient does not awaken from irreversible brain injury.

Talk to Her involves two male–female relationships, with both female characters in persistent vegetative state (PVS). The management of and recovery from PVS is pivotal in this film. The title of the film refers to talking to a patient in PVS. Major topics are discussed in this film, and all are incorrectly depicted. Cinematically, the film is considered by many film critics a career highlight for Almodóvar, known for high melodrama, operatics, and vivid colors, but neurologically it is problematic. Early in the movie, we are introduced to one of the patients (4 years in PVS) showing no contractures, perfectly toned and tanned body, eyes closed, mouth slightly open, with a hint of a smile. I named this cinematic portrayal the "Sleeping Beauty phenomenon" (Figure 3.1).

Quotable Lines of Dialogue

Talk to Her	
Friends of patients to each other	*Why are you so sure she does not hear you?*
	Because her brain is turned off.
Physician	*Is there hope? No. I repeat, scientifically no, but if you choose to believe, go ahead.*

Screenwriters should be told by neurologists that patients in a vegetative state lack awareness, have no purposeful behavior, and have marked muscle bulk loss, severe contractures despite the best rehabilitation efforts, high risk of decubital ulcers, sepsis, and major medical complications. To be fair, this film nonetheless shows the meticulous care given to the patients, with clean sheets being provided as well as a tracheostomy and gastrostomy. (For neurology purists, the tracheostomy is usually removed shortly after successful weaning.) Foot splints to help in avoiding contractures are shown as well as the application of eye drops.

In the film, one of the PVS patients becomes pregnant, and the male nurse is convicted of rape. This introduces another new, complex medical

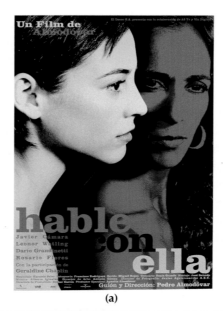

(a)

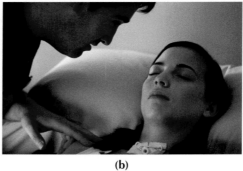

(b)

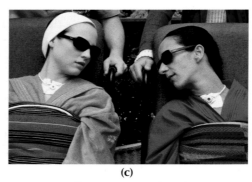

(c)

FIGURE 3.1 (a) Actors in *Talk to Her*. (Used with permission of El Deseo Da S.L.U photo; Miguel Bracho.) (b) Note features of "Sleeping Beauty phenomenon." (c) Two patients with tracheostomies.

problem that is inaccurate. Pregnancy in PVS patients is physiologically not likely. Most stop menstrual cycles, and even in patients who are pregnant and become vegetative, fetal loss is substantial. In this movie, for dramatic purposes, the pregnancy is brought to term and the woman delivers a stillborn baby.

A PVS is diagnosed when the patient has a severe—often devastating—brain injury with no awakening since onset. Gradually, the patient starts opening eyes ("eye open" coma), and sleep–wake cycles start. Patients may grimace, but there is no sign of awareness of self or what is happening at the bedside (no response to family members, no response to nursing staff or physicians). The patient just breathes, may yawn or clench the jaw, and may have some startle head movements (particularly to loud sounds), but is mute except for occasional sounds. The patient has "vegetative" symptoms, meaning an intact autonomic nervous system (blood pressure, heart rate, and respiratory function fluctuate). The facial features change dramatically, and the patient becomes unrecognizable to family members if they visit weeks later. (A perfect cinematic example is in *The Descendents* [2011], covered in Chapter 4.) Contractures occur; decubital wounds are unavoidable and may need treatment. Patients are very vulnerable to infections. There is no evidence of suffering. Recovery is not expected after a year in this situation (mostly when injury is due to prior cardiac arrest, traumatic brain injury, or both).

Some films suggest reading to the patient in prolonged coma (*Rocky II*, 1979), even suggesting it could reduce the time in coma (*Uptown Girls*, 2003), but this is not based on fact. In the movies, some coma patients in film may shed tears. In reality, many patients in a PVS shed tears spontaneously and it is neither a sign of awareness nor a sign that improvement is possible. Shedding tears has been used most dramatically and misleadingly in *The Past* (2013). Although the physician forcefully argues it is not an accepted stimulus, the husband of a comatose woman tries to elicit a reaction using her perfumes (he claims that smell is the last of the senses to disappear). After he sprinkles himself with perfume, he leans over the patient and she sheds a tear, which he does not see, standing at the opposite side of the bed. She does not squeeze his hand when asked. (In an interview, the director explained that his intention was to show a subtle response that is often not recognized, and because it is not recognized a decision may be made to withdraw support.) The use of perfume is notable here, because it has been used in (unproven) coma stimulation programs.

Similarly of interest is *The Dreamlife of Angels* (1998) ⁀⁀⁀ which also depicts a comatose patient with contractures, tracheostomy, and gastrostomy remarkably well. Several patients are shown with contractures and nurses using gastrostomy for feeding. It also shows attempts by nurses to record eye tracking and fixating on an object by the comatose patient— often a first sign of improvement.

In *Firelight* (1997) ⁀⁀, a reasonably good representation is given with eyes open, coma, and contractures, but again the facial features continue to be unaffected in this movie portrayal, and the patient has a doll-like appearance.

Prognosis is a common theme in films showing PVS, and screenwriters have used terms such as "the garden" (nursing home) and "vegetable" (PVS). In *Blind Horizon* (2003), the physician prognosticates: "50% total recovery, 35% partial, and 15% you plant him in the ground and watch him grow." The most recent film on coma is *Dormant Beauty*, 2012, ⁀ loosely based on the famous PVS case in Italy (Eluana Englaro). The film unfortunately does not provide any insights into this cause célèbre.

We have studied the use of coma by screenwriters in great detail. Movies on coma were reviewed for cause and situation of coma, demographics of actor in coma, physician communication of coma, awakening from coma, and the role of the neurologist. Some representative films are shown in Table 3.1. Because there is violence in R-rated movies, coma was typically caused by motor vehicle accidents, gunshot wounds, and other violent causes. Most actors were in their 30s to 40s. A review of 30 movies with coma portrayal showed awakening in 60%, including time in coma up to 10 years.

Successful rehabilitation after many years of coma was also shown, mostly with full physical and cognitive recovery. After awakening, murderous revenge was common, as seen in *Lying in Wait* (2001), *A Man Apart* (2003), *Face/Off* (1997), and *Hard to Kill* (1990).

Awakening was often seen after a bizarre trigger (smoke, mosquito bite, sudden bright sunlight). In *While You Were Sleeping* (1995), the actor awakens during a New Year's Eve party after having been "comatose" for most of the film.

Most gratuitous is a scene in *Good Bye Lenin!* (2003) ⁀, where a comatose mother awakens after 8 months on a ventilator when her son enters the room, flirts with the nurse, and kisses her. Inexplicably, his mother is immediately lucid upon awakening. Other awakenings have showed a confused patient fighting with nursing staff or pulling out intravenous

TABLE 3.1 Examples of Coma in Fiction Film

Year	Title	Rated	Director	Plot	Actor Portraying Coma	Cause
1979	*Rocky II*	PG	Sylvester Stallone	Love motivation	Talia Shire	Hemorrhage in pregnancy
1983	*The Dead Zone*	R	David Cronenberg	Psychic	Christopher Walken	MVA
1990	*Hard To Kill*	R	Bruce Malmuth	Revenge	Steven Segal	GSW
1993	*Short Cuts*	R	Robert Altman	Loving family	Lane Cassidy	MVA
1995	*While You Were Sleeping*	PG	Jon Turteltaub	Love; loving family	Peter Gallagher	Accident
1997	*Face/Off*	R	John Woo	Revenge	Nicolas Cage	Violence
1997	*Firelight*	R	William Nicholson	End-of-life decisions; murder to be with another woman	Uncredited	Accident
1997	*Winterschläfer (Winter Sleepers)*	NR	Tom Tykwer	Loss, grief	Uncredited	MVA
1998	*Seven Hours to Judgment*	R	Beau Bridges	Revenge	Uncredited	Violence
2001	*The Safety of Objects*	R	Rose Troche	End-of-life decision	Uncredited	MVA
2002	*28 Days Later*	R	Danny Boyle	Changed world; escaped killer virus	Gillian Murphy	MVA
2002	*Swim Fan*	PG-13	John Polson	Attempted murder	Monroe Mann	MVA
2003	*Kill Bill: Vol. 1*	R	Quentin Tarantino	Revenge	Uma Thurman	GSW
2003	*Blind Horizon*	R	Michael Haussman	Coma causes amnesia	Val Kilmer	GSW
2003	*A Man Apart*	R	Gary Gray	Revenge	Vin Diesel	Violence
2004	*Paparazzi*	PG-13	Paul Abascal	Revenge	Uncredited	MVA

Note: MVA: motor vehicle accident; GSW: gunshot wound; PG: parental guidance; NR: not rated, R: restricted lines, as if awakening from a nightmare. Awakenings have also included suddenly sitting upright in bed (*Kill Bill: Vol. 1*); sudden awakenings with stepping out of bed, pulling out catheters, and walking out of the hospital (*28 Days Later*); and sudden increase in pulse rate before awakening (*While You Were Sleeping* [1995], *Face/Off* [1997]). True to its title, in *Hard to Kill* (1990), Steven Segal has been in coma for many years and has grown a sizable beard. During the "awakening scene," he relives the violent assault to him and his family just before he opens his eyes. His heartbeat is up; he grunts from anger, then opens his eyes and looks stunned.

One must to conclude from these observations that screenwriters markedly deviate from current accepted knowledge. More importantly, we were interested to learn how this was perceived by the audience. We proceeded to use 22 key scenes from 17 movies to show a group representing the lay public. These 72 viewers were asked to use statements to rate for accuracy, such as:

"I think this is how comatose patients look."

"I think the awakening shown after being in a coma for a long time can happen this way."

"After awakening from being in a coma for a long period of time, you may be able to do this."

"I believe what has been said is correct."

"If my family member would be in the same situation, it is possible that I would remember what happened in the scene and allow it to influence any decisions that I would make."

The survey results are shown in Figure 3.2. Viewers were unable to identify important inaccuracies in one-third of the selected scenes, and one-third of the viewers expressed that these scenes could influence decisions if they would be in a similar situation. This result suggests that movies may have a considerable impact on the public's perception of coma (although two-thirds did not think any of it was accurate). Similar findings were seen with a small sample of non-neurology residents, but not with neurology residents, who could identify all inaccuracies (unpublished observations by Wijdicks).

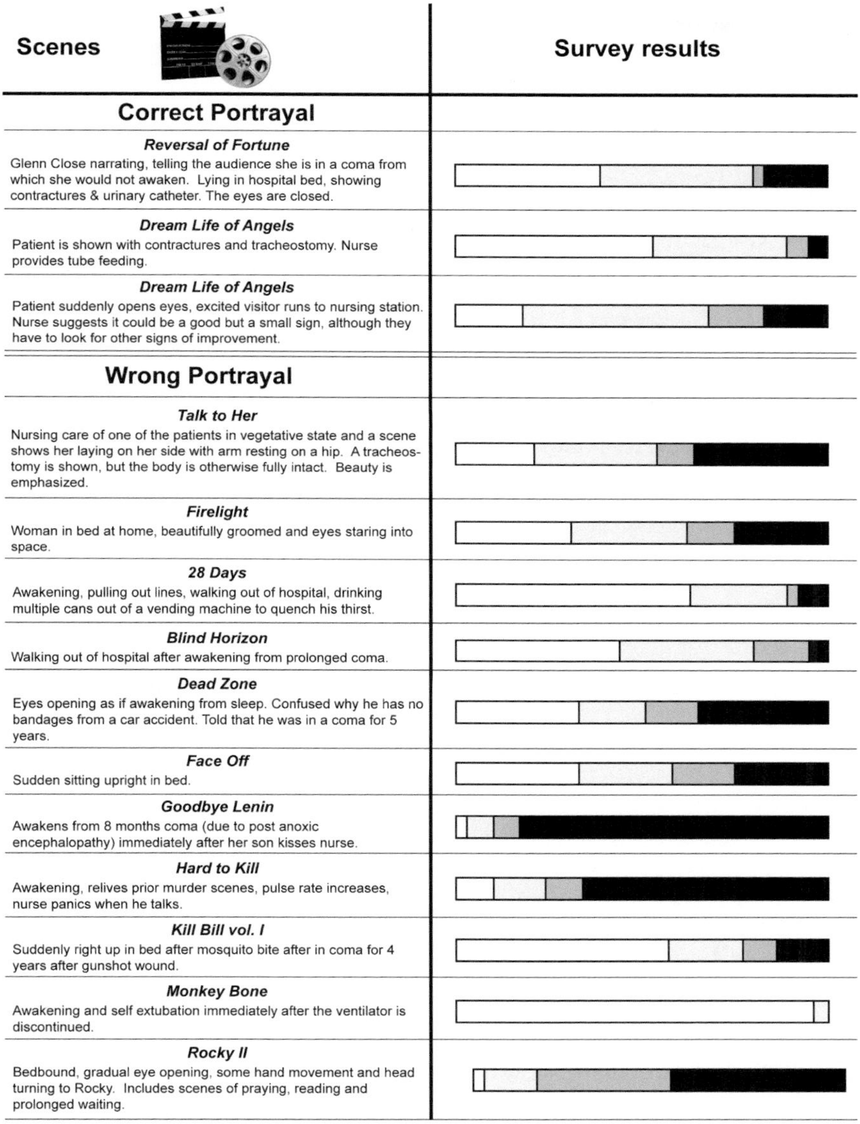

Scenes	Survey results

Correct Portrayal

Reversal of Fortune
Glenn Close narrating, telling the audience she is in a coma from which she would not awaken. Lying in hospital bed, showing contractures & urinary catheter. The eyes are closed.

Dream Life of Angels
Patient is shown with contractures and tracheostomy. Nurse provides tube feeding.

Dream Life of Angels
Patient suddenly opens eyes, excited visitor runs to nursing station. Nurse suggests it could be a good but a small sign, although they have to look for other signs of improvement.

Wrong Portrayal

Talk to Her
Nursing care of one of the patients in vegetative state and a scene shows her laying on her side with arm resting on a hip. A tracheostomy is shown, but the body is otherwise fully intact. Beauty is emphasized.

Firelight
Woman in bed at home, beautifully groomed and eyes staring into space.

28 Days
Awakening, pulling out lines, walking out of hospital, drinking multiple cans out of a vending machine to quench his thirst.

Blind Horizon
Walking out of hospital after awakening from prolonged coma.

Dead Zone
Eyes opening as if awakening from sleep. Confused why he has no bandages from a car accident. Told that he was in a coma for 5 years.

Face Off
Sudden sitting upright in bed.

Goodbye Lenin
Awakens from 8 months coma (due to post anoxic encephalopathy) immediately after her son kisses nurse.

Hard to Kill
Awakening, relives prior murder scenes, pulse rate increases, nurse panics when he talks.

Kill Bill vol. I
Suddenly right up in bed after mosquito bite after in coma for 4 years after gunshot wound.

Monkey Bone
Awakening and self extubation immediately after the ventilator is discontinued.

Rocky II
Bedbound, gradual eye opening, some hand movement and head turning to Rocky. Includes scenes of praying, reading and prolonged waiting.

(a)

FIGURE 3.2 Key scenes and accuracy ratings of viewers with no medical expertise.

Scenes	Survey results

Dead Zone
Neck brace, crutches, and trying to walk ten steps after 5 years in coma.

Kill Bill vol. I
Immediately after awakening, patient goes out of the hospital in wheelchair. She is unable to move her legs, but uses her arms.

Talk to Her
Walking with cane and no visible scars or long term effects after awakening from vegetative state.

Uptown Girls
Nanny: "You can read out loud." Daughter: "He is a vegetable." Nanny: "I saw this show on TV once with all these sick people, and the ones with the families that talked to them held on 10 times longer than the ones that were left alone, and that is a fact."

Regarding Henry
"He is driving, just went off the side of the road. Doctor says forget it, no chance. Three months later, he beat me in tennis. Swear to God, you never know...you never know."

Lying in Wait
"What was it like being in a coma?
You can hear everything, but you can't wake up so you wait and wait and start thinking...the first thing that comes to mind is food, then you think about sex, the women you had, the women you wanted to have..."

Critical Care
Conflict between daughter of comatose patient and physician. Daughter suggests the patient can hear her and understands questions. Physician's interpretation is it is hard to tell.

Critical Care
Physician assistant repeatedly tries to convince tapping of the comatose patient's finger is a Morse code (patient was a signal man in the Navy) and finds out it means "if you love me."

Legend: Correct assessment | Somewhat correct assessment | Neutral | Somewhat incorrect assessment | Incorrect assessment

(b)

FIGURE 3.2 (*Continued*)

A Final Word

Several well-known feature films include an actor in coma and show actors as a "sleeping beauty." Trivializing coma to a sleeplike state is totally inaccurate and potentially problematic. These films also show awakening, but never accurately, and the scenes as written are highly improbable. Awakening is gradual and slow and not infrequently as if awakening from a nightmare. Seldom do directors and screenwriters use information in a meaningful way or correctly convey the major consequences of coma and rehabilitation. Prolonged comatose states in the movies are misrepresented. We found that the general viewer is capable of identifying these inaccuracies, but a substantial minority is fooled by such depictions. Do screenwriters have a responsibility to be cautious? I think so.

Further Reading

Bernat JL. Chronic disorders of consciousness. *Lancet* 2006;367:1181–92.

Monti MM, Vanhaudenhuyse A, Coleman MR, et al. Willful modulation of brain activity in disorders of consciousness. *N Engl J Med* 2010;362:579–89.

Mosberg WH, Jr. Trauma, television, movies, and misinformation. *Neurosurgery* 1981;8:756–58.

Wijdicks EFM. The bare essentials: Coma. *Practical Neurology* 2010;10:51–60.

Wijdicks EFM. *The Comatose Patient.* 2nd ed. New York: Oxford University Press, 2014.

Wijdicks EFM, Cranford RE. Clinical diagnosis of prolonged states of impaired consciousness in adults. *Mayo Clin Proc* 2005;80:1037–46.

Wijdicks EFM, Wijdicks CA. The portrayal of coma in contemporary motion pictures. *Neurology* 2006;66:1300–3.

TRAUMATIC BRAIN INJURY IN FILM

Regarding Henry (1991); starring Harrison Ford, Annette Bening, and Bill Nunn; directed by Mike Nichols, written by Jeffrey Abrams; distributed by Paramount Pictures.

Rating

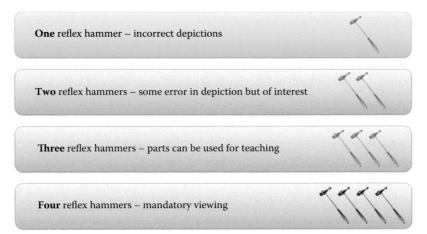

One reflex hammer – incorrect depictions

Two reflex hammers – some error in depiction but of interest

Three reflex hammers – parts can be used for teaching

Four reflex hammers – mandatory viewing

The Lookout (1991); starring Joseph Gordon-Levitt, Jeff Daniels, and Matthew Goode; written and directed by Scott Frank; best first feature at Independent Spirit Awards; distributed by Miramax Films.

Rating

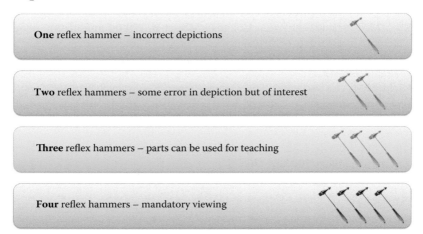

One reflex hammer – incorrect depictions

Two reflex hammers – some error in depiction but of interest

Three reflex hammers – parts can be used for teaching

Four reflex hammers – mandatory viewing

Criticism and Context

Regarding Henry is considered one of the most recognizable movies about the long-term effects of severe traumatic brain injury (TBI). This movie is about a callous, arrogant attorney who gets shot in the head while getting cigarettes late at night. He is resuscitated from blood loss, causing additional anoxic injury. (The movie surprisingly suggests that he could do well if it only had been a gunshot to the right side of the brain.) In several scenes we see him, following a neurosurgical procedure, remaining comatose for some time. There is uncertainty about his prognosis. Then he suddenly opens his eyes but does not fixate and remains mute.

Quotable Lines of Dialogue

Regarding Henry	
Physician	*Mrs. Turner, your husband is incredibly lucky. The bullet wound to the head caused minimal damage. See, it hit the right frontal lobe. That's the only part of the brain that has redundant systems. I mean, if you're going to get shot in the head, that's the way to do it.*
Colleague attorney	*… and went off the side of the road. The doctor says forget it, no change. Three months later he beat me in tennis, swear to God, you never know … you never know.*

The film shows the long, painful rehabilitation and recovery from traumatic brain injury well. ("It is going to be a long, tough rehabilitation." "The brain is very mysterious." "In some ways he is starting from scratch here.") After he seems to be improving and returns home, the film shows him markedly changed. In one scene, Henry is wandering the street buying a hot dog (he does not know what "'kraut" is), answering a phone in a random phone booth, watching an X-rated movie, and buying a puppy—all in one afternoon.

Regarding Henry is, of course, about redemption—learning to start anew, being a better person with a blank slate after prolonged coma. Initially, the personality changes after such an injury that are depicted here are very real. Frontal lobe injuries result in major problems in mood (the flat mimicry of Harrison Ford is generally accurate), difficulty understanding complete conversations, and loss of verbal fluency. Henry also shows impulsivity and disinhibition so common after these types of injuries. However, the "clean slate," and even more, the change to a lovable person in this film is far less likely because most patients remain easily irritable or their prior personality flaws become accentuated. These types of brain injuries do not make a person a better being; the person is changed forever and must cope with major attentional deficits and emotional lability.

Another notable film—at least for a couple of opening scenes—is *The Lookout*. This film has some interesting things to say about the long-term consequences of TBI. Chris (Joseph Gordon-Levitt) is injured in a motor vehicle accident (MVA), and we see him later explaining his difficulty with "sequencing"—putting things he does during the day in order. He cannot remember names. He writes down exactly how his day is planned and who he meets, and then follows this routine. He meets his female case manager, and there are some sexual innuendos. ("Did you have these thoughts before head injury?") There are yellow notes everywhere, multiple notebooks, and drawers with names for clothing. He also unhinged quickly and has a "frontal" behavior. He shares a room with a jokester blind man (Jeff Daniels), who he can turn to if he forgets how to open a can. The movie turns into a caper involving a bank heist, and there is little further explanation of his behavior. One of the reasons the screenwriter wrote this character is that Chris seems subdued and thus oblivious to his surroundings. *The Lookout* is a generally accurate representation of the "forgetfulness" of patients with moderate TBI. The inability to organize the day ("sequencing") does occur, and using Post-it notes on telephones as a reminder to call someone is a credible behavior. Many patients work with compensatory strategies, and cognitive rehabilitation may improve the executive aspects of attention and everyday functioning. Memory strategy training has also been developed, and includes notebooks to compensate for deficits. Electronic memory aids using reminder messages often meet needs.

Trauma (2003) ⌐ also concentrates on "recovery" from an MVA. Colin Firth is briefly comatose but awakens. He has full flashbacks of the entire accident when looking at pictures of his wife (who died in the accident), feels people are looking at him, startles easily, and hallucinates. The psychologist or psychiatrist (not credited) explains these episodes. ("It is not uncommon especially when you are tired… that it [the brain] translates sounds or sights into images of that.") He visits old friends, who tell him, "Get on with your life." The film shows a posttraumatic stress disorder well, but soon it becomes clear that the film belongs more in the horror genre.

The most recent film on traumatic brain injury can probably be ignored. *Post Concussion* (1999) ⌐ is a comedy about a person with a concussion who is unable to go back to work and has a lot of headaches. He is tested for personality and recall. He has a virtually impossible line to repeat: "Though they had bad disguises, it was their inscrutable style that allowed them to escape the dogged policemen." Then he is blindfolded and performs a round-hole test. The narrator comments that "the medical profession does not understand the psychological ones." After these tests, he is declared unfit for work. There are black-and-white inserts in which a scientist pokes in a cow's brain to explain a concussion and personality disorders. There is little substance in this film; testing of brain-injured patients is ridiculed, and there is much to object to—and it is not funny, either.

A Final Word

No shortage of trauma and gunshots in the entertainment industry—no poetic realism here. In the early days of Hollywood, the depiction of head injury had already started in Westerns, with scenes showing bar fights and people getting hit on the head by a poker (or a chair or a bar stool). Head injury is common in the movies, but it is remarkable that the effects of traumatic head injury are rarely shown. There are some good teachable scenes in these films, but also questionable ones. Readers of this book who are looking for accuracy are better off viewing *The Crash Reel* (2013), discussed in detail in Chapter 5.

Further Reading

Azouvi P, Vallat-Azouvi C, Belmont A. Cognitive deficits after traumatic coma. *Prog Brain Res* 2009;177:89–110.

Cicerone KD, Langenbahn DM, Braden C, et al. Evidence-based cognitive rehabilitation: Updated review of the literature from 2003 through 2008. *Arch Phys Med Rehabil* 2011;92:519–30.

Fleminger S. Long-term psychiatric disorders after traumatic brain injury. *Eur J Anaesthesiol Suppl* 2008;42:123–30.

Lewis FD, Horn GJ. Traumatic brain injury: Analysis of functional deficits and posthospital rehabilitation outcomes. *J Spec Oper Med* 2013;13:56–61.

Powell LE, Glang A, Ettel D. Systematic assessment and instruction of assistive technology for cognition (ATC) following brain injury: An introduction. *Perspectives on Neurophysiology and Neurogenic Speech and Language Disorders* 2013;23:59–68.

Stuss DT. Traumatic brain injury: Relation to executive dysfunction and the frontal lobes. *Curr Opin Neurol* 2011;24:584–89.

Warriner EM, Velikonja D. Psychiatric disturbances after traumatic brain injury: Neurobehavioral and personality changes. *Curr Psychiatry Rep* 2006;8:73–80.

STROKE IN FILM

Amour (2012); starring Jean-Louis Trintignant, Emmanuelle Riva, and Isabelle Huppert; written and directed by Michael Haneke; received Palme d'Or Award at Cannes Film Festival, César Award for best film, Academy Award for best foreign language film, among many US and international nominations; distributed by Artificial Eye and Sony Pictures Classics.

Rating

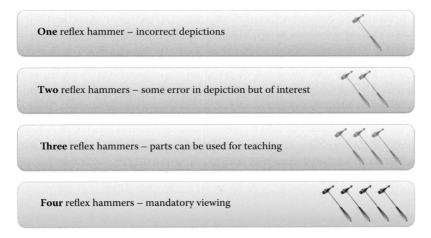

One reflex hammer – incorrect depictions

Two reflex hammers – some error in depiction but of interest

Three reflex hammers – parts can be used for teaching

Four reflex hammers – mandatory viewing

A Simple Life (2012); starring Andy Lau, Deanie Ip, and Fuli Wang; directed by Ann Hui, written by Susan Chan; Volpi Cup for best actress at Venice Film Festival, among other Asian film festival awards; distributed by Distribution Workshop.

Rating

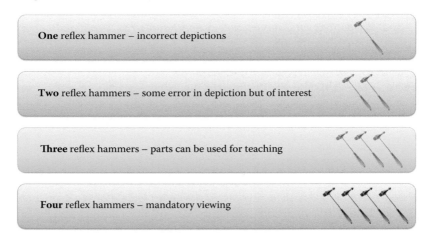

One reflex hammer – incorrect depictions

Two reflex hammers – some error in depiction but of interest

Three reflex hammers – parts can be used for teaching

Four reflex hammers – mandatory viewing

Criticism and Context

Amour is a brilliantly directed film by Michael Haneke about the life-changing effects of a stroke in the nearest and dearest. *Amour* is one great lovely touch and changes one's outlook on the topic. *Amour* is a character study of two highly cultivated octogenarian piano teachers, Anne (Emmanuelle Riva) and Georges (Jean-Louis Trintignant), and their daughter Eva (Isabelle Huppert), played phenomenally by three icons of French cinema. The film is quiet, staged as classic theater, and filled with emotional dialogue mixed with Schubert's impromptus. Haneke, a luminary of cinema, is known for films that show life as it is. Many of us can identify with his characters. Haneke forces us to not only watch the scenes, but also to witness the events and feel the heaviness of being in compromising situations. Arguably, he does this without manipulating the audience. The idea for the *Amour* screenplay came from Haneke's personal experience helplessly watching an elderly family member deteriorate from frailty and commit suicide.

Anne suddenly develops neurologic symptoms, is devastated by a stroke, and deteriorates. Georges is now faced with the care of his wife. Initially, this seems not too much of a chore, but soon things change as the care becomes increasingly complex.

Amour offers some clues on Anne's condition, but there is little to allow a detailed neurologic assessment. In an indelible scene, the sudden speech arrest and frozen stare—with no recollection—is dramatic (Figure 3.3) and closest to what appears to be a complex partial seizure. She subsequently has difficulty pouring tea using her right hand. A major blockage in her carotid artery is found, followed by vascular surgery (endarterectomy), and she is left with profound right-sided weakness but no speech impediment. She is wheelchair bound. Before surgery they have been told she could have a 5% chance of complications; but apparently she does not belong to the supposedly 95% risk-free surgical group. There is no doctor–patient conversation about the complication, which seems to be treated as a matter of fact and just bad luck—a classic Haneke theme.

Quotable Lines of Dialogue

Amour	
Georges	*What can I say? The carotid artery was blocked. They did an ultrasound scan, two in fact, and they said they had to operate on her. She was confused and scared.... They said the risk was very low and that if they didn't operate, she'd be certain to have a serious stroke.*
Eva	*And what do they say now?*
Georges	*Just that it didn't go well. It's one of the 5% that go wrong.*

Soon after this surgery, Anne develops another, far more devastating stroke. This should give pause to any neurologist. Stroke specialists—assuming the first presentation was a stroke and not a seizure or an unclear spell with asymptomatic carotid disease—may certainly come away with some reservations if (at least in this film) the result is much worse than before and quickly leads to another stroke. Carotid endarterectomy has been performed in octogenarians, and vascular surgeons have reported no increase in postoperative mortality or stroke when compared with "younger" patients. Carotid endarterectomy may be justified knowing the average life span of a woman of 85 years is still about 5 years; and thus there might be the, albeit unproven, potential for benefit. All of this may not terribly relevant to the main plotline of the movie, but it could prompt discussion about medical and surgical decisions in the vulnerable very old. Coercion into questionable surgery after a questionable event with eventually poor results could easily be another frightening theme for Haneke.

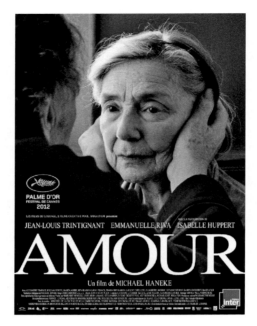

FIGURE 3.3   Film poster of *Amour* showing the key scene of Anne's sudden stare associated with speech arrest. (Used with permission of El Deseo Da S.L.U photo; Miguel Bracho.)

Emmanuelle Riva is unsurpassed as playing a stroke victim, and there is truly no better representation on film. Georges, played just as convincingly by Jean-Louis Trintignant, nurtures her to the best of his ability, though he is hampered by his own frailty. He provides for all transfers, performs passive range of motion, and even provides melodic intonation therapy. There is some humor in this part of the film, and it is very touching to see both Anne and Georges try to make the best of the situation. Together they look at photos from earlier times, eliciting Anne's response, "It is beautiful…this long life."

But now they seem imprisoned in their Paris apartment. The only contact with the outside world is a concerned neighbor (and a pigeon). Professional support at this stage would have been expected, but Georges has little except for a biweekly visit with a family doctor, who tells Georges that admission to the hospital after the second stroke would have little use and staying home would spare her all these tests. Also, Anne told him clearly that she would never want to be hospitalized again. She rejects any form of sympathy and gets visually irritated when the topic comes up. Georges displays repressed pain, and by the time his exhaustion becomes visible, he fires a private nurse. He tells his alienated daughter, "None of this deserves to be shown."

A major element of the film is the loneliness but also the desire to be left alone, even if assistance is offered. This might be one of the main lingering themes for neurologists to consider: How do we organize care for stroke patients after they are dismissed from the hospital, and can we help and improve their dignity? Do we appreciate the spouse's ordeal and offer assistance?

Amour is not specifically about how society deals with the problems or infirmities of the elderly, but the film could still start that discussion. All of this cannot be waved away as if it could only happen in France (or Europe), because it can happen anywhere, and to anyone. In a very dramatic way, the film shows the familiar, yet often unrecognized, problems of denial and burnout in a caregiver. At the end of life, the ultimate sign of love may be to provide relief of pain and suffering, which the movie shockingly portrays after Anne has signaled refusal of fluids and frequently cries out in pain. Is this the crime of passion of advanced age?

Amour shows us the cruel change in a loving relationship brought about by illness. The realization that genuine, deeply rooted love for each other is the only thing we have and that it may be suddenly taken away for no good reason, just at random and unannounced, is painful to watch. It also sheds a harsh light on the major problems with the home care of a neurologically disabled patient; I cringed each time Anne with her swallowing difficulties was given water and coughed. The lack of adequate neuropalliation is very apparent and a warning. *Amour* is an unforgettable work of art.

A similar theme has recently been explored in the film *A Simple Life*, this time in Hong Kong. Ah Tao (played by Deanie Ip) suffers a nondominant hemispheric stroke. She suddenly develops a left-sided hemiparesis and dysarthria, portrayed very well. Her "master" (as she calls him), Roger (Andy Lau), is not allowed to care for her, and she wants to go to a nursing home. Her main motivation is that she knows a second stroke is coming and that this is the end of it. She refuses to be cared for and prefers a drab nursing home. Roger now feels responsible for her well-being (Ah Tao worked 60 years for his family), and his normal daily routine changes, visiting her frequently and just trying not to neglect her. Ah Tao tries to hold on to her dignity. The film has been somewhat overshadowed by the grandeur of *Amour*, but this work is equally important in depicting a new reality after a major stroke. There is full recovery, and the film does emphasize changing relationships and compassion, but it does not provide any more insight in management of a stroke. The title refers to a simple life, and that is what is shown.

Stroke has been rarely depicted in film. Equally memorable (discussed in the next section) is *The Diving Bell and the Butterfly* (2007), which is an extreme manifestation of what appears to be an acute clot in the basilar artery. Some films—*Legends of the Fall* (1994) ⌃ and *Flawless* (1999) ⌃— explore stroke, but they do not deal with the human toll on relationships. Moreover, these two films show stroke portrayed in a curious way by world-class actors. Robert De Niro plays a character with marked dysarthria and crooked smile in *Flawless* (1999) and Anthony Hopkins plays a character who suffers a stroke in *Legends of the Fall* (1994). Hopkins contorts his face to one side, moans and groans, but is able to write full words on a chalkboard hanging on his neck. He is also able, in the climactic shootout scene, to kill everyone using his paralyzed side. *Run & Jump* 2014 ⌃ depicts bilateral frontal lobe infarcts and is chosen by the director to depict behavior problems. How the family copes with this condition is insufficiently developed. Conor (Edward MacLiam) is more sullen than parkinsonian, more hesitant than aphasic, and more childish than inappropriate, but then again how do you play such an extremely rare and far more serious condition? In these films, other than showing a turn for the worse, dealing with adversity, and suddenly being hit by a major handicap, there is no further insight or explanation about stroke in the screenplay.

A Final Word

Observing the rapid neurologic decline of a loved one is unfathomable. These films focus on one major aspect of humanity—the desire to engage in and maintain loving relationships when such an ordeal strikes. When you see *Amour*, I am sure it will force you to ask these questions: Are we doing enough to prevent this isolation in couples? How might we better help them accept the reality? What are the consequences of certain medical care choices? *Amour* and *A Simple Life* do not answer these questions—they do not have to do that—but they will have the viewers think about it - for quite some time.

Further Reading

Cecil R, Thompson K, Parahoo K, McCaughan E. Towards an understanding of the lives of families affected by stroke: A qualitative study of home carers. *J Adv Nurs* 2013;69:1761–70.

Greenwood N, Mackenzie A, Cloud GC, Wilson N. Informal primary carers of stroke survivors living at home—Challenges, satisfactions and coping: A systematic review of qualitative studies. *Disabil Rehabil* 2009;31:337–51.

Langhorne P, Bernhardt J, Kwakkel G. Stroke rehabilitation. *Lancet* 2011;377: 1693–1702.

Ski C, O'Connell B. Stroke: The increasing complexity of carer needs. *J Neurosci Nurs* 2007;39:172–79.

LOCKED-IN SYNDROME IN FILM

The Diving Bell and the Butterfly (Le scaphandre et le papillon) (2007); starring Mathieu Amalric, Emmanuelle Seigner, Marie-Josée Croze, Anne Consigny, and Max von Sydow; directed by Julian Schnabel, written by Ronald Harwood; best director award at the Cannes Film Festival, Golden Globe Award for best foreign language film, César Awards for best actor and best editing; distributed by Pathé and Miramax Films.

Rating

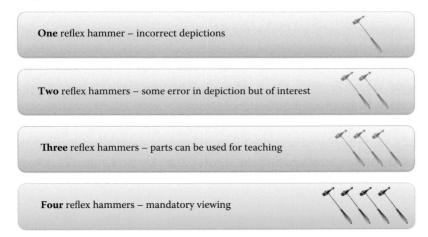

One reflex hammer – incorrect depictions

Two reflex hammers – some error in depiction but of interest

Three reflex hammers – parts can be used for teaching

Four reflex hammers – mandatory viewing

Criticism and Context

The Diving Bell and the Butterfly is based on an autobiography "written" (blinked) by Jean-Dominique Bauby (*Le scaphandre et le papillon*). Bauby, as played by Mathieu Amalric, was editor-in-chief of the fashion magazine *Elle* when he had a stroke at the age of 43 years. The cause is unknown but, in this age group, most likely was a vertebral artery dissection with basilar artery occlusion (or, less likely, a pontine hemorrhage from an arteriovenous malformation). The locked-in syndrome makes it impossible for the patient to move, and only eye movement (eyelid blinking and up and down eye movements) is possible. There is no effective swallowing, and patients initially need assistance with ventilation. Vision, hearing, and feeling are all preserved. Here the mind is truly locked in a nonfunctioning body.

The director, Julian Schnabel, appropriately decided to make the movie in French. In an interview with Charlie Rose, Schnabel explained that he made the movie after his father died, as a self-help device to help himself deal with his own inevitable death. The film is accurate and unique in showing Jean-Dominique as what he would have seen in this condition. On the screen, Jean-Dominique's visual field is shown through the lens of the camera. Blinking is imitated by having the cinematographer move objects in front of the camera. His thoughts are the main narrative in the film. The camera shows double vision, difficulty focusing, and a constricted keyhole visual field, which would be quite correct if—in the setting of a basilar artery occlusion—the posterior occipital fields were involved. It also mostly shows his limitation of eye movements, although the camera does move vertically and horizontally and scans the room. (In locked-in syndrome, only vertical eye movements are possible, which then would produce double vision.) Nonetheless, it remains highly speculative what patients see in the acute phase. The rehabilitation and extreme effort of a speech therapist to communicate with him are notable and mostly correct. Standard orientation questions are asked ("Are we in Paris?" "Does wood float?"). In patients with locked-in syndrome, establishing communication is, however, far more difficult in the early poststroke phase, although later computer-assisted communication can be very effective.

It clearly shows an important technique of communicating, starting with the alphabet, using the most commonly used letters (all attempts start with the letter E). Jean-Dominique was able to dictate a full work (Figure 3.4) but died soon after its publication. Jean-Dominique felt like he was living in a diving bell and could use his memory and imagination to go to past worlds (thus the butterfly feeling). "My cocoon becomes less oppressive and my mind takes flight like a butterfly."

The movie includes a forceful scene when he dictates, "I want to die," creating a negative, overly dramatized reaction to the speech therapist; but according to the real transcriber, this was never mentioned (nor was

she present during his demise, in contrast to what was shown in the film).
Bauby's case is unique, and his book has given us insight into the condition.

Quotable Lines of Dialogue

The Diving Bell and the Butterfly	
Dr. Lepage (neurologist)	*It won't comfort you to know that your condition is extremely rare.… We simply do not know the cause.… I'm afraid it's just one of those things.*
Dr. Lepage	*You've had what we call a cerebrovascular accident. It's put your brain stem out of action. The brain stem is an essential component of our internal computer. In the past, we would have said you'd had a massive stroke. You would very probably have died. But now we have such improved resuscitation techniques that we're able to prolong life.*
Bauby	*I do want to die. I really do.*
Speech therapist	*That makes me very angry. There are people who love you and care for you. I'm a complete stranger and yet I care for you. And you're alive. So, don't say you want to die. It's offensive. It's… it's obscene.*

One of the most existential fears is being trapped in one's own body and being misdiagnosed as comatose. In 1844, Alexandre Dumas described such a state in the fictional character of Monsieur Noirtier, who was in this condition for more than 6 years and was described as a "corpse with living eyes." Ironically, as an aside, Jean-Dominique noted in his book that he wanted to write a book based on Dumas's *The Count of Monte Cristo* before this ordeal.

Improved communication and meticulous care may lead to some prolongation of survival and even acceptable quality of life. However, a far more insightful book is by historian Tony Judt, *The Memory Chalet*, where he describes his decline from ALS (amyotrophic lateral sclerosis) and becoming locked in. His book is, in his own words, "nostalgic recollections of happier days." His description of his affliction is "… and there I lie; trussed, myopic and motionless like a modern-day mummy alone in my corporeal prison accompanied for the rest of the night only by my thoughts."

The locked-in syndrome is a major deafferentation syndrome sparing hearing, vertical eye movement, blinking sensation, and pain perception.

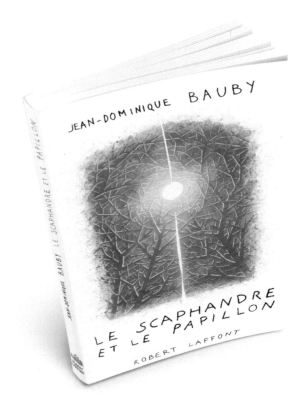

FIGURE 3.4   First edition of Bauby's book. Bauby blinked more than 200,000 times to produce this 137-page book describing his desolate state before he died. (Used with permission of Robert Laffont.)

It has been rarely transient, but patients with so-called *locked-in syndrome plus* syndrome (some arm preservation) can improve fairly dramatically over time. The film correctly identifies improvement of oropharyngeal function as a potential prelude to recovery of speech. Paralysis remains virtually always profound, as is the imbalance, creating major rehabilitation difficulties.

A Final Word

The Diving Bell and the Butterfly is one of the iconic films in this *Neurocinema* collection and should be required viewing for any physician. There are lessons to be learned about how to best communicate with patients, the power of communicating with respiratory therapists, and the tremendous challenge of rehabilitation. Late recovery has not been reported, but patients may remain cognitively intact for years. Some improvement may occur, such as movement of fingers, which allows better signaling. A large proportion of patients die from pulmonary complications—and it seems Bauby's fate as well—but some have survived for many decades. Studies have suggested that some patients may have reasonably acceptable days despite being trapped in an immobilized body, but only if best care and compassion can be provided for a prolonged time. Maximal compensatory auditory and visual stimulation are required to compensate for the loss of other senses. With a feat of great willpower.

Further Reading

Burki T. In the blink of an eye. *The Lancet Neurology* 2008;7:127.

De Massari D, Ruf CA, Furdea A, et al. Brain communication in the locked-in state. *Brain* 2013;136:1989–2000.

Goldberg C, Topp S, Hopkins C. The locked-in syndrome: Posterior stroke in the ED. *Am J Emerg Med* 2013;31:1294 e1291–93.

Mathiasen H. Mind over body: The diving bell and the butterfly. *Am J Med* 2008;121:829.

Ohry A. The locked-in syndrome and related states. *Paraplegia* 1990;28:73–75.

Phipps E. A view from the inside: The diving bell and the butterfly. *J Head Trauma Rehabil* 1999;14:89–90.

Snoeys L, Vanhoof G, Manders E. Living with locked-in syndrome: An explorative study on health care situation, communication and quality of life. *Disabil Rehabil* 2013;35:713–18.

BRAIN TUMOR IN FILM

Dark Victory (1939); starring Bette Davis, George Brent, Humphrey Bogart, Geraldine Fitzgerald, and Ronald Reagan; directed by Edmund Goulding, written by Casey Robinson, based on the play by George Brewer Jr. and Bertram Bloch; multiple nominations, including best director at the Academy Awards, but no wins; distributed by Warner Brothers.

Rating

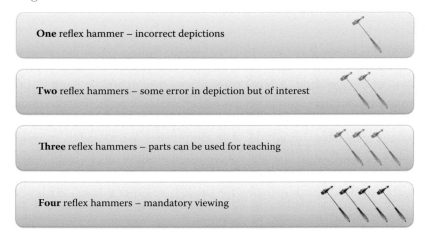

Declaration of War (*La Guerre est déclarée*) (2011); starring Valérie Donzelli, Jérémie Elkaïm, César Desseix, and Gabriel Elkaïm; directed by Valérie Donzelli, written by Valérie Donzelli and Jérémie Elkaïm; distributed by IFC Films.

Rating

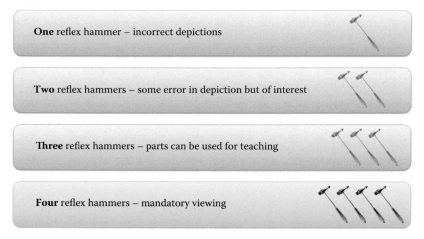

Criticism and Context

Two key films—dramatically different in approach and accuracy—deserve detailed discussion.

Dark Victory is a farce when it comes to neurologic manifestations of a brain tumor. The protagonist gets headaches after some sort of aggravation, develops sudden double vision, and falls off a horse but still refuses to see a doctor. ("He will say it is a hangover and I am smoking too many cigarettes.") She then notices burns on her right hand. She sees a neurosurgeon, and he asks, "Does the light bother you? How did you play at bridge?" He then proceeds with summarizing her problem: "Progressive headache for months, vision is cut in half just as if someone is shutting folding doors, that queer feeling in your right arm—you cannot laugh that off.... Your memory is shot to pieces. You cannot concentrate." The neurologic exam is shown. "Please squeeze my hand." He tests reflexes (normal) and sensory testing (alternating the use of a piece of silk and a rough cloth). After this exam, he consults three other physicians and tells her to proceed with surgery for brain tumor. When he discovers that the tumor is malignant, he still tells her that there will be "complete surgical recovery."

Quotable Lines of Dialogue

Dark Victory	
Neurosurgeon	*Technically it is called glioma.*
Patient	*Sounds like a plant.*
Neurosurgeon	*Yes, it is like a plant—a parasitic one.*
Friend	*How will it come?*
Neurosurgeon	*Peacefully, God's last small mercy.*

Dark Victory, which I suspect is known by few neurologists as a major motion picture on the presentation of a brain tumor, is bold because it addresses the dilemma of how to discuss the diagnosis. Clinical presentation of a malignant brain tumor can be nondistinctive. It is usually of recent onset over days rather than months and may be a change in pattern in a patient with prior headaches. Nausea and vomiting are common (but rarely seen in film). Seizures are presenting symptoms in up to 40% of patients and are often focal rather than generalized. Personality changes are also common.

After surgery, she demonstrates good walking (even demonstrates walking backwards and tests her own reflexes). When her brain tumor recurs, it presents as diminished vision ("getting dark," hence the title), becoming blind. It all happens within minutes. She says goodbye to her dogs, unsteadily climbs the stairs, goes to bed, and dies peacefully. *Dark*

Victory contains scenes giving misleading information and highly unusual clinical presentation. Nothing can even be attributed to the zeitgeist of the times.

A much better film is the autobiographical *Declaration of War*. The directors and their child play the lead roles. It was even filmed in the same hospital where they had this similar experience. The film is, therefore—albeit somewhat fictionalized—reasonably precise, certainly when it comes to the medical and neurologic aspects. Romeo and Juliette are their fictional names, and their child (Adam) does not seem to thrive at the age of 3 and then has difficulty walking and vomits. A facial asymmetry is noticed. This leads to multiple physician contacts, but they use largely ambiguous language that confuses everybody. The parental stress is enormous, and the contact with physicians is rough and distanced. At one point, Romeo says to Juliette, "No outsmarting the doctors, no idiotic theories, no Internet."

Quotable Lines of Dialogue

Declaration of War	
Parents	*Are there possible aftereffects?*
Neurosurgeon	*There must not be any.*
Parents	*But if there are?*
Neurosurgeon	*There will be no aftereffects. (Puts hands on mother's shoulder.) Get some rest. Don't count eggs in the hen's ass. Sleep well. See you tomorrow.*

The movie is about how this experience could change parents of a very sick child. It is a must-see film for pediatric neurologists and residents. There are family frictions, strangers who have an opinion, irritations in the hospital, extreme financial burden (even in "free healthcare Europe") and their marriage does not end well. The narrator says, "They stopped working for 2 years. They separated, got back together several times, and then separated for good. Each started a new life." The end shows a final visit with their (this time) compassionate neurosurgeon; and, when seen 5 years later, the child is cured. The war is won.

The film is useful because of several neurologic aspects. First, the presentation that "something might be wrong" and the delay to come to a final diagnosis in a young child are not uncommon. In children less than 2 years old, behavioral changes, seizures, vomiting, and head tilt are common (and nonspecific). Not infrequently, only one-third of the children are diagnosed within one month of onset of presentation due to a doctor's delay but also parental delay. The film does inappropriately show the neurologist vacillating on outcome with a general pessimistic outlook. Concerning, however, is the presentation of a tumor diagnosed as "rhabdoid." It will not be apparent to most viewers and even general neurologists, but atypical teratoid rhabdoid tumors are very aggressive, with high mortality in the first year. It would be very unusual to survive disease free from this diagnosis. (A "10%" survival is mentioned here and even that may be too optimistic.) Ifosfamide carboplatin and etoposide (ICE) treatment is mentioned (a common approach in Europe, and different in the United States, where methotrexate and high-dose chemotherapy and stem cell rescue is considered).

Some other lesser-known films deserve mention. In the Dutch movie *Turkish Delight* (1973) ⁘, one of the most accomplished works of Paul Verhoeven, the protagonist, Olga (Monique van de Ven), is diagnosed with a brain tumor after she loses concentration at her work (bottles fall off the conveyor belt). She is then found unresponsive, and in the next scene, crying in the middle of a pneumoencephalogram procedure. She displays infantile and aggressive behavior. A nurse runs in to give her sedative drugs. ("Bad, bad Missus. What are we? Wild and naughty.") In a deeply sad ending she dies the next morning. Again, there is a misrepresentation here of wild psychotic behavior in a patient with a newly diagnosed brain tumor. A scene showing (now obsolete) pneumoencephalography is one of the most memorable shocking moments in this film.

Another film that portrays brain tumor in detail is *Crisis* (1950) ⁙. In *Crisis*, the Hopkins neurosurgeon Dr. Ferguson (Cary Grant) is asked to see the dictator Raoul Farrago, who is presenting with a left temporal lobe meningioma. He needs surgery, but the outcome is uncertain. ("Can he live without surgery? Not much chance. Can he live after surgery? I do not know.") Dr. Ferguson is advised to leave the country and not get involved, and is even advised to kill him in surgery. ("When you have the president with his head open…one little slip of the knife…then who will know?") He proceeds with surgery and seems to recover well, but the dictator dies from postoperative hemorrhaging after he defends himself against a revolt.

Brain tumor, and finding a cure, is a theme in Aronofsky's *The Fountain* (2006), but it does not present much detail on diagnosis or management, and it is purely fantastical. *Phenomenon* (1996) is about a brain tumor causing new powers instead of deficits and is discussed separately in Chapter 6.

A Final Word

The diagnosis of a malignant brain tumor—little time to live—is a major theme in a considerable number of films. Coping with childhood tumors has rarely been depicted successfully in the movies. The surgery, chemotherapy, and physician interaction are all depicted very well in *Declaration of War*. This film is the best representation of brain tumor in children in film, and has a happy ending. *Dark Victory* is a classic but not because of its neurological representation. Withholding important medical information, or worse, sharing medical details (and prognosis) with others and not the patient should be vexing for many physicians, and these are perhaps the most stunning aspects of *Dark Victory*.

Further Reading

Crawford J. Childhood brain tumors. *Pediatr Rev* 2013;34:63–78.
Dobrovoljac M, Hengartner H, Boltshauser E, Grotzer MA. Delay in the diagnosis of paediatric brain tumours. *Eur J Pediatr* 2002;161:663–67.
Epelman S. The adolescent and young adult with cancer: State of the art—Brain tumor. *Curr Oncol Rep* 2013;15:308–16.
Huttner A. Overview of primary brain tumors: Pathologic classification, epidemiology, molecular biology, and prognostic markers. *Hematol Oncol Clin North Am* 2012;26:715–32.
Omuro A, DeAngelis LM. Glioblastoma and other malignant gliomas: A clinical review. *JAMA* 2013;310:1842–50.

MENINGITIS IN FILM

The Courageous Dr. Christian (1940); starring Jean Hersholt, Dorothy Lovett, and Robert Baldwin; directed by Bernard Vorhaus, written by Ring Lardner Jr. and Ian McLellan Hunter; distributed by Stephens-Lang Productions.

Rating

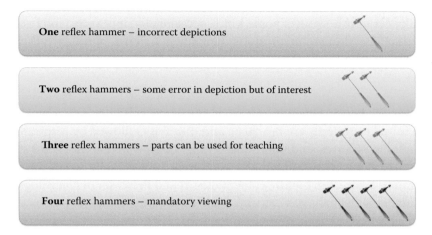

In Enemy Hands* (2004); starring William Macy, Til Schweiger, and Thomas Kretschmann; directed by Tony Giglio; distributed by Lions Gate Entertainment.

Rating

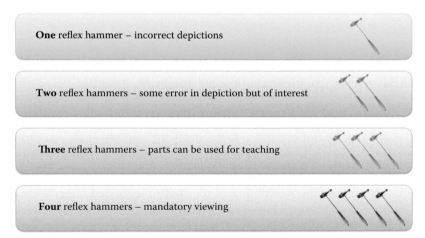

Criticism and Context

It may be surprising that so few films deal with meningitis, and only with outbreaks. The main difficulty for screenwriters, I suppose, is that meningitis is just one illness and one person, and it is definitively more sweeping when it affects and kills many and does so rapidly. Such outbreaks (usually a virus of some kind) occasionally appear as Hollywood themes. The ultimate medical disaster movie about a prevalent virus is *Contagion* (2011), directed by Steven Soderbergh. The fictional virus MEV-1 is a mix of bat and pig virus ("somewhere the wrong bat met up with the wrong pig") and is modeled after the Nipah virus outbreak of April 1999 in Malaysia, when 265 cases of febrile encephalitis were reported. The initial symptoms are headache and dizziness followed by respiratory symptoms, seizures, and rapid-onset coma. *Contagion* does not show specific neurologic manifestations or neurologic involvement except for one terminal seizure. Ian Lipkin, epidemiologist and Professor of Neurology at Columbia University was consulted and devised the imaginary virus and built a clinical scenario of such an epidemic. The film asks the important questions of how the public health organizations would respond in such a disaster scenario and how quickly vaccines would be developed.

The spread of the virus shown in *Contagion* is very similar to the H1N1 virus epidemic that infected people in more than 40 countries. The film correctly points out that in future epidemics there will be massive challenges to the rapid manufacture of vaccines.

Infectious outbreak was on display in the summer blockbuster zombie movie *World War Z* (2013). In this movie, parasite manipulation of the collective behavior of ants—a concept rooted in actual science and ant behavior—is used to induce host discrimination in the zombies. The "manipulated" zombies then selectively choose to infect only healthy hosts but refrain from infecting the terminally ill. Brad Pitt's own infection with Ebola virus protects him. Within the context of the story, this raises the preposterous prospect of protecting people by infecting them with some deadly but curable disease until the zombie epidemic abates. Another virus (simian virus ALZ-113) is used to exterminate the world's population with very few survivors (*Dawn of the Planet of the Apes,* 2014).

Apart from the otherworldliness of the above-mentioned films, there are two interesting movies on meningitis outbreaks. *The Courageous Dr. Christian* is one of several movies made about the character Dr. Christian in the late 1930s and early 1940s. Dr. Christian is an eminent country doctor played by the Danish actor Jean Hersholt. It is rumored that the actor's demeanor as a kind and knowledgeable doctor resulted in mail sent to him by viewers asking for advice.

This movie, set at the end of the Depression, has as its major theme an epidemic of meningitis. The meningitis epidemic outbreak apparently starts in "Squatter Town," a section of town with poor sanitation. The people—the poor and the needy—are a constant concern ("people living around the bend"), and the city board decides to remove them. It finally comes to a major confrontation between Dr. Christian and the police.

Quotable Lines of Dialogue

The Courageous Dr. Christian	
Dr. Christian	*Chief, there is a child in here with spinal meningitis.*
Chief	*That does not sound serious to me, doctor.... It is just a stall.*
Dr. Christian	*It is a highly contagious disease with high mortality rate.*
	A single case may rapidly spread over the whole district.
Mayor	*This meningitis is just a kid disease, isn't it?*
Dr. Christian	*Hardly, it hits all ages and classes.*

The film shows a child who is sensitive to light and sound and who cries easily (Mother: "Don't be such a crybaby"), but Dr. Christian (stroking his chin while looking serious) thinks the child may have meningitis. He performs a lumbar puncture, and the film shows him finding the characteristic inflammatory polynucleated cells under the microscope. The mayor asks if it is only the "squatters," but Dr. Christian—irritated by the lack of compassion for the poor—tells him the infection may also get to the town administrators.

Dr. Christian orders everybody to be inoculated, and he creates makeshift hospitals. Newspaper headlines are shown. "Crisis Looms. Disease Getting Beyond Control." Multiple people on gurneys are shown, but there soon is a break with no new cases, a decline in the number of cases, and improvement in the condition of patients.

Most likely, the outbreak in *The Courageous Dr. Christian* represented meningococcal meningitis, as major American cities in the early 1900s were hit by these epidemics. (The meningococcus bacterium was identified in 1905 by Simon Flexner.) The film accurately mentions treatment with sulfa drugs and the use of serotherapy (administration of meningococcal horse antiserum). Epidemic meningitis was a major concern in the United States, particularly in a country mobilized for war. The first randomized trial involved nearly 14,000 men of the US Army basic training centers, and the polysaccharide vaccine proved to be safe, with a 90% reduction in cases.

Throughout the world, meningococcal meningitis remains a formidable problem (0.5 cases per 100,000 in the United States, but 10–1,000 per 100,000 in Africa). Meningitis epidemics caused by meningococcal disease are seen in one-third to two-thirds of infected persons, with sepsis in 30% of the cases resulting in hypotension and intravascular coagulation (causing petechiae and purpura). The disorder—if survived—leads to major disability, including hearing loss, seizures, and spasticity. These outbreaks may lead to rapid demise of large numbers of children, and recent outbreaks in the Western world are still observed. Every outbreak is met with alarm, and therefore such a response is accurately depicted in this film.

Another film with meningitis as a plot driver is *In Enemy Hands*. The film is primarily a story involving a US Navy submarine in World War II. The movie names, for the first time, the diagnosis meningococcal meningitis. One of the crew members starts coughing, then detects a rash, and starts vomiting later. The medic—although not sure—suggests meningococcal meningitis, but due to patient refusal is unable to quarantine the man, who soon dies. The boat gets torpedoed by the Germans, and they abandon ship only to be rescued by the German crew. There the US captain has the same symptoms but decides not to tell. "Keep it between you and me. I do not want to startle the crew." Soon eight members fall ill. One of the crew members recognizes the rash because his sister had it and died in 7 days. Soon the whole boat is coughing, but the outbreak gets little further attention or is worked out. Nonetheless, the environment where the epidemic emerges is well chosen. Many of these epidemics occurred in military barracks and college dorms, and vaccination is now mandatory.

Two films show a scene with a missed diagnosis of meningitis. In *The Men* (1950), one of the traumatic spine injury patients develops fever. It shows testing for neck stiffness, a lumbar puncture, and the surgeon in charge going bonkers after the patient dies. The movie *Barbara* (2012) also shows a missed diagnosis of meningitis. Barbara (played by Nina Hoss) is a physician sent to a small sea town in north East Germany close to the Baltic Sea. A girl is admitted, confused and belligerent. The physician prepares for a sedative because she apparently had been admitted many times with fake diseases. (It is later revealed that she is in a hard-labor camp and tries to escape using fake medical illness as an excuse.) Barbara discovers neck stiffness and proceeds with a lumbar puncture. Apparently the girl had hidden in the woods in an attempt to escape, and tick-borne meningoencephalitis is diagnosed. It realistically shows that meningoen-cephalitis can present with behavior problems and requires vigilance. The patient recovers after she is treated with "serum." This is a quite timely scene, particularly because tick-borne encephalitis is prevalent in Eastern Europe and Russia and in the summer. Most cases at the time were seen in Germany, and the areas formerly known as Czechoslovakia and the USSR. The incubation time is a median 8 days after a tick bite. The mentioned "serum treatment" is unexplained because there is no specific treatment for tick-borne encephalitis, only prevention by active immunization.

A Final Word

Infections of the central nervous system are only of interest to filmmakers when an epidemic with panic and alarm is involved. Rapid death is more often shown than coma or seizures. Sporadically, a case of meningitis is introduced, but only to show that the disorder is not recognized or not diagnosed by physicians. Some scenes (*Barbara*, 2012) can be lifted for educational purposes because the representation is accurate (for example, showing neurologic examination for neck stiffness).

Further Reading

Artenstein AW, LaForce FM. Critical episodes in the understanding and control of epidemic meningococcal meningitis. *Vaccine* 2012;30:4701–7.

Bernstein R. Science on set. *Cell* 2013;154:949–50.

Flexner S, Jobling JW. Serum treatment of epidemic cerebro-spinal meningitis. *J Exp Med* 1908;10:141–203.

Halperin SA, Bettinger JA, Greenwood B, et al. The changing and dynamic epidemiology of meningococcal disease. *Vaccine* 2012;30 Suppl 2:B26–36.

Lindquist L, Vapalahti O. Tick-borne encephalitis. *Lancet* 2008;371:1861–71.

Lipkin WI. The real threat of *Contagion*. *The New York Times*. September 11, 2011.

Shah S. Viral disaster movie. *Lancet* 2011;378:1211.

Stephens DS, Greenwood B, Brandtzaeg P. Epidemic meningitis, meningococcae-mia, and *Neisseria meningitidis*. *Lancet* 2007;369:2196–2210.

ENCEPHALITIS LETHARGICA IN FILM

Awakenings (1990); starring Robert De Niro and Robin Williams; directed by Penny Marshall, written by Steven Zaillian; nominated for multiple Academy Awards but won best actor (Robert De Niro) at the New York Film Critics Circle Awards; distributed by Columbia Pictures.

Rating

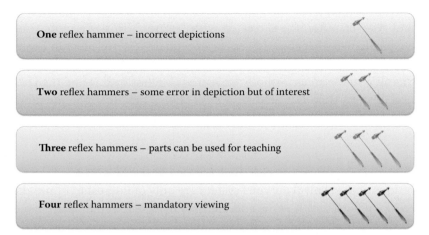

One reflex hammer – incorrect depictions

Two reflex hammers – some error in depiction but of interest

Three reflex hammers – parts can be used for teaching

Four reflex hammers – mandatory viewing

Criticism and Context

Encephalitis lethargica debuted in Vienna in the winter of 1916–1917. Constantin von Economo, to whom identification of the disorder is credited, described cases that were seen in a psychiatry ward. The infection became intermittently pandemic through 1918 throughout Europe and the United States. The cause (presumably a virus) has never been identified, and such an outbreak—as an epidemic of this proportion—has not returned. There is a misunderstanding that this disorder was caused by the major influenza epidemic, also known as the Spanish flu, during the final year of the Great War (1918). In his paper (Figure 3.5), von Economo suggested that the responsible lesion was a sleep-promoting area in the hypothalamus, and indeed sleep could be induced in animal studies later after lesioning these areas.

Awakenings is centered upon Leonard Lowe (Robert De Niro), who is afflicted with encephalitis lethargica and then has a miraculous improvement, but only temporarily. Robin Williams plays Oliver Sacks as Dr Sayer with all the mannerisms and aloofness of a befuddled neuroscientist (Chapter 2). The patients are all in a frozen, immobile (catatonic) state, but Dr. Sayer—much to the surprise of the staff—shows they can catch a ball, catch a dropping pen, and respond to music. After Leonard improves dramatically, all of the other patients improve immediately on L-dopa, turning a sedate institution into a lively place. This over-the-top presentation has been criticized, but the portrayal of parkinsonism is quite correct, including the later dystonic movements.

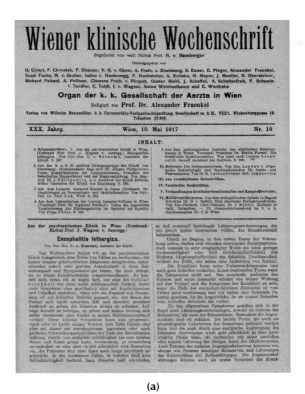

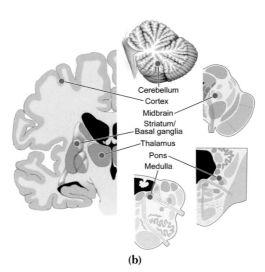

Cerebellum
Cortex
Midbrain
Striatum/
Basal ganglia
Thalamus
Pons
Medulla

(b)

FIGURE 3.5   (a) Title page of the article on encephalitis lethargica by Constantin von Economo. (b) Drawing showing the widespread lesions not only in the midbrain and thalamus, which produces the "lethargica," but also in other parts of the brain.

What is currently known about the disorder is that patients with encephalitis lethargica—after a flu-like illness—develop, marked sleepiness, ocular movement disturbances, and fever. Abnormal posturing (dystonia) was not initially part of the manifestation, and stupor (hence the word lethargic) was most prominent and persistent. Some patients could become immediately alert; others had more cyclic responsiveness, with sleep during the day and wakefulness during the night. According to earlier descriptions, paralysis of eye muscles was very common, but very often, other cranial nerves were involved. Oropharyngeal dysfunction could lead to early demise. This combination of upper cranial nerve involvement and stupor now, in retrospect, would fit well with an upper brainstem lesion and, indeed, the mesencephalon showed necrosis and perivascular lymphocytic infiltrate. In some patients, the hypothalamus was involved. Many of these patients either developed a catatonic state or recovered with narcolepsy. The parkinsonian manifestations occurred often after a period of time, even years after the infection, but more than 50% of the survivors developed parkinsonian symptoms in 5 years and 80% in 10 years. Oculogyric crisis was a common manifestation.

No treatment was available for these excessively sleeping patients. Oliver Sacks remembers he originally planned a 3-month double-blind clinical trial of L-dopa in institutionalized patients with parkinsonism and stupor from encephalitis lethargica; this was prompted by earlier work on the use of aromatic amino acids in improving parkinsonism. Nine cases improved greatly. That became the basis of the main manuscript, which was initially rejected by several medical and neurologic journals, but was published in 1972 in *The Listener* under the title "The Great Awakening." Later, with 11 more case histories, the book *Awakenings* was published, which was the inspiration of this movie. Oliver Sacks described his observations in *Awakenings* as follows: "These 'extinct volcanoes' erupted into life.… occurring before us was a cataclysm of almost geological proportions, the explosive 'awakening,' the 'quickening,' of eighty or more patients who had long been regarded, and regarded themselves, as effectively dead."

Quotable Lines of Dialogue

Awakenings	
Leonard's mother	*I do not understand it. He was never any trouble before. He was good, quiet and obedient.*
Dr. Sayer	*Because he was catatonic, Mrs. Lowe.*

Awakenings (continued)

Dr. Sayer, in conversation with Dr. Ingham	*What must it be like to be them? What are they thinking?*
	They are not. The virus didn't spare the higher faculties.
	We know that for a fact?
	Yes because the alternative would be unthinkable.

According to Vilensky's extensive review of the subject, encephalitis lethargica was significantly overdiagnosed despite being distinct enough to be recognized. *Awakenings* focuses on postencephalitis Parkinson's disease, but the syndrome as described by von Economo could present as meningitis, predominant ophthalmoparesis (oculomotor and abducens), and increasing somnolence to deep stupor.

It is fascinating that still new cases of encephalitis lethargica are diagnosed, and some have described children with basal ganglia encephalitis. N-methyl-D-aspartate antibodies were found in 10 of 20 patients with encephalitis lethargica, which would suggest it may be an autoimmune encephalitis and, more importantly, that it may respond to immunotherapy. Many of these patients (young females) have dystonic movements involving face and arms.

A Final Word

Awakenings is often the first movie that comes to mind when neurologic portrayal in the movies is discussed. It is sometimes even used—mistakenly—in lectures on coma. The movie may, however, imply that "comatose patients," after 20 years, could awaken with a simple drug administration. Not everyone was pleased with this film, and the seemingly haphazard administration of L-dopa—as depicted in the film with secretly doubling the dose despite the serious side effects—led two bioethicists to use this as an example of an unethical drug trial, in particular in a disabled vulnerable population. This is unfair not only because one cannot use current standards for clinical trials for a study done 40 years ago, but also because the original study was carefully performed.

The overlap with the Spanish influenza epidemic has always been intriguing, and some cases of influenza may have been misdiagnosed as encephalitis lethargica. When postencephalitic parkinsonism appeared, it presented with a catatonia (frozen in a certain position). Facial expressions disappeared, and very often upward involuntary eye movements (oculogyric crises) occurred. Rigidity was common, but tremor—as is typical in Parkinson's disease—was not. The number of patients who developed postencephalitic Parkinson's disease was small, albeit there were hundreds of descriptions. This episode was a significant period in the history of neurology, and sufficient proof of concept has been established.

Further Reading

Dale RC, Church AJ, Surtees RA, et al. Encephalitis lethargica syndrome: 20 new cases and evidence of basal ganglia autoimmunity. *Brain* 2004;127:21–33.

Dale RC, Irani SR, Brilot F, et al. N-methyl-D-aspartate receptor antibodies in pediatric dyskinetic encephalitis lethargica. *Ann Neurol* 2009;66:704–9.

Holt WL, Jr. Epidemic encephalitis: A follow-up study of 266 cases. *Archives of Neurology & Psychiatry* 1937;38:1135–44.

Sacks OW. *Awakenings*. London: Picador, 1982.

Sacks OW. The origin of *Awakenings*. *Br Med J (Clin Res Ed)* 1983;287:1968–69.

Sacks OW, Kohl M, Schwartz W, Messeloff C. Side-effects of L-dopa in postencephalic parkinsonism. *Lancet* 1970;1:1006.

Vilensky J. *Encephalitis lethargica: During and after the epidemic*. New York: Oxford University Press, 2011.

von Economo C. Encephalitis lethargica. *Wiener Klinische Wochenschrift* 1917;30:581–85.

Wolitz R, Grady C. Use of experimental therapies. In: *The Picture of Health: Medical Ethics and the Movies*. Colt H, Quadrelli S, Friedman L (eds.). New York: Oxford University Press, 2011.

SPINAL CORD INJURY IN FILM

The Intouchables (2011); starring François Cluzet, Omar Sy, and Anne Le Ny; written and directed by Olivier Nakache and Éric Toledano; César Award for best actor (Omar Sy) as well as many other major US and international nominations; distributed by Gaumont Film Company.

Rating

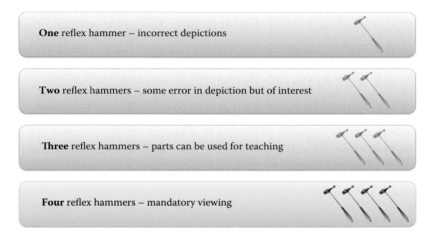

One reflex hammer – incorrect depictions

Two reflex hammers – some error in depiction but of interest

Three reflex hammers – parts can be used for teaching

Four reflex hammers – mandatory viewing

Criticism and Context

Acute traumatic spinal cord injury immediately and disastrously changes a person's life. When it occurs, it is most common in young active males (in their late teens and twenties), mostly from car crashes, and in some, as a result of hazardous winter sports, after a flash of foolishness such as diving off a rock into shallow water (*The Sea Inside*, Chapter 4), the use of trampolines, and as a result of violence or extreme circumstances such as war.

The lauded film—and unprecedented European box-office hit—*The Intouchables* (based on a true story) describes in great detail the physical care and emotional challenges of a well-to-do aristocrat, Philippe (François Cluzet), with acute high cervical cord injury after a paragliding crash. Paragliding was his favorite form of recreation because he felt grandiose and was on top of the world ("he felt he could pee on the world"). Philippe—a man of means—has a plethora of caregivers. Omar Sy plays the Senegalese Driss, who incidentally has a criminal record and spent 6 months in jail for robbery. Philippe decides to hire Driss in part because Driss doesn't show him any pity and because the other caregivers are humorless and boring.

The film suggests that the wealthy may have a better deal when it comes to such a dramatic handicap, and it all seems quite droll. Nonetheless, the film provides some unique insights and is very well researched. In showing the burdens of a quadriplegic person, no film before has provided such detail for the audience. Driss is portrayed here as an ignoramus laughing about major pieces of art and music. He is most satisfied when he hears the motor of a Philippe's Maserati roar and when he can dance to his own favorite music. The film is about two fully dependent persons—one on full medical support, the other on government money. In a key conversation, Philippe says, "You don't mind living off others' backs?" and Driss pointedly answers, "No, how about you?"

A bothersome scene is when Driss discovers Philippe does not feel the hot silver teapot and then pours a little more of potentially scalding tea on his legs until another caregiver interrupts. Another notable scene is the "hyperventilation" attacks as a result of "phantom pain." There is also one episode that suggests painful cramping due to spasticity. This results in Driss taking him out in the early Paris hours, where he explains his problems with control of these excruciating attacks. During another attack, Driss decides to give him a joint, and the film clearly suggests that marijuana might be a therapeutic option. They seemed to have a great time using marijuana. This is problematic territory, particularly as addiction is more common in patients with severe spinal cord injury and chronic pain.

Quotable Lines of Dialogue

The Intouchables

Philippe	*The medication has its limits.… Doctors call them phantom pains. I feel like a frozen steak tossed onto a red-hot griddle. I feel nothing but suffer anyway.*

The film admirably brings out the major problem of pain management in patients with acute spinal cord injury. Pain after a spinal cord injury is a dull musculoskeletal joint ache or dull abdominal pain, but the most pain is the one generated centrally. Allodynia is common (pain with simple touch), but so is hyperalgesia. Spontaneous sharp, shooting, unrelenting pain often described by the patient as a feeling of hot stabbing knives may occur and may be resistant to medication. Surgical approaches (dorsal root entry zone lesioning, or cordomyelotomy) are often insufficient, and there are varying results with transcutaneous electrical nerve stimulation.

The film discusses manual fecal removal, and Driss's refusal. ("I don't go for this sick stuff.") The film appropriately discusses bowel dysfunction because most reflex activity below the level of spinal cord injury is lost. Defecation in patients with cervical cord lesions requires the diaphragmatic contraction because the abdominal muscles required for straining are lost. Constipation is common, with some incontinence. Manual evacuation and digital stimulation in combination with mini-enemas is commonly used, and some patients with chronic obstruction may need a colostomy.

Problems with sexuality are also prominently mentioned in this film, and sex through erogenic zones is discussed. Psychogenic arousal requires thoracolumbar spinal cord function and thus is absent. In spinal cord injury, males may have reflex erections but no orgasms or ejaculation. Patients often discover that nipples, earlobes, or inner thighs evoke genital awareness, and men can experience orgasms despite absent erections.

The film hints at mortality, and the protagonist mentions his shortened life expectancy. It correctly implies that cervical injury at 50 years will have a mortality of 30% in 20 years (threefold higher than a healthy person). Complications are directly related to immobilization and associated with infections such as urosepsis, respiratory failure, pulmonary embolus, and increasing risks of renal stones and pressure sores, but there is also the uncomfortable issue of suicides.

Philippe has a scar from a tracheostomy, which is accurate considering the level of cord injury he has suffered. The phrenic nerve, which innervates the diaphragm, originates from the C4 spinal segment, with some contributions from C3 and C5. Patients with a C3/C4 lesion—as in Philippe—will likely be ventilator dependent; and equally so, patients with a C5 lesion are far more likely to be liberated successfully. The abdominal component to breathing—mostly coughing up—is lost due to absent tone in paralyzed muscles. Many of these patients visibly use their accessory (sternocleidomastoid and scalene) muscles to assist in respiration. Philippe's breathing in the film does not seem to be compromised at all. Often only short sentences can be spoken with deep inhalations in between and use of accessory muscles. For the filmmaker, it must have been too much of an additional downer to show all that.

The Intouchables is a complex film on the challenges of being paralyzed from the neck down and an important addition to the collection of *Neurocinema*. The credits of *The Intouchables* say that 5% of the profits from the film was donated to the Association Simon de Cyrène in Paris, whose purpose is to create shared living spaces for disabled adults and friends. Something really good came out of this financial blockbuster movie.

Another major film, based on the true story of skier Jill Kinmont, is *The Other Side of the Mountain* (1975) ⚞ starring Marilyn Hassett and Beau Bridges, which correctly depicts the challenges of living with a cervical spine injury. The confrontation of the physician with parents is telling. ("All we can do is hope." "Hope that she will walk?" "No, hope that she will live.") She remains wheelchair bound, and the movie focuses on toughness and doing away with self-pity and an "anything can be overcome" theme. (Parenthetically, the film shows her best friend, crippled by polio, chastising her not to be so self-centered and to try to find a way to live with this handicap.) She becomes a successful teacher, but not after being confronted with prejudice. ("People think that when your toes are numb your brain is numb." "Paraplegics are unacceptable as teachers in this country.") Even in this prim and proper tearjerker, making love and having no feeling is discussed. ("You want more than me; you get tired of it.")

Paraplegia is a far more common topic in cinema than quadriplegia, and there are numerous actors playing paraplegics. A major distinction should be made between amputees and paraplegics. Amputees are better rehabilitated, and often a transition to better lives is shown in the movies after wearing prostheses (recall Gary Sinise as Lieutenant Dan in *Forrest Gump* [1994] and, more recently, Marion Cotillard as Stephanie in *Rust and Bone* [2012]).

Acute paraplegia in film often involves coping and not coping. Most films simply show the rejection by others and the threat of isolation, but a few provide fresh insight into the changed circumstances of the patient with paraplegia.

Quotable Lines of Dialogue

The Men	
Doctor	*In almost every case, the word "walk" must be forgotten. It no longer exists.*
Mother	*My boy is only 19.*
Doctor	*But with proper care he may live to be 90.*
Doctor	*The legs are gone now. The head has to take over.*

The most important film in this regard is *The Men* (1950) ⚞, which mostly handles how couples can adjust to their lives. It is Marlon Brando's debut playing an introvert-depressed paraplegic. The film was shot in Birmingham Veterans Administration Hospital in Van Nuys, California (close to Hollywood), and included a cast of actual patients. A key scene comes early in the movie when the crass prima donna, Dr. Brock, explains (in the hospital's chapel) to spouses of affected veterans that this is a lasting injury. Living with a paraplegic is an overarching theme in this film. It also daringly—noting the year it was filmed—approaches not only the topic of sexuality ("I am not a man; I cannot make a woman happy.") but also fertility ("It is not very probable but in the realm of possibility."). Even Bud's in-laws weigh in ("Is it so wrong for us to want a grandchild?"). Bud marries but returns to the hospital after a spat. Several times, during stressful moments, he jerks his right leg to—reasonably correct—imitate spasms.

Many legendary filmmakers have used paraplegia in war casualties to point out—in their view—deficiencies in care of the disabled. One perspective is in *Born on the Fourth of July* (1989) ⁀, an indictment of the Veterans Affairs (VA) hospitals—this time the Bronx Veterans Hospital—with horrendous display of medical care of T7 paraplegic Ron Kovic, played by Tom Cruise. The representation of the VA hospital is a dirty, unorganized cesspool with rats crawling under the beds. Cynicism is rampant when, in the morning, the nurse calls, "Everybody rise and shine." When Ron asks a doctor if he will be able to have children, he answers resolutely, "No, but we have a very good psychologist here." Massive decubitus is seen, and patients seem to be lined up for "group defecation." Ron is allowed to walk with crutches without help in a show of alpha male behavior, but falls and fractures his leg. The care at home is frustrating, and acceptance is nonexistent. Ron Kovic is left alone with poor skin and bladder care and lack of any compassion.

Similar situations of life after war-related Vietnam spinal cord injury are found in *Coming Home* (1978) ⁀⁀⁀. The film also shows a deplorable hospital with paraplegics in the Vietnam war era. There is urine spilling over after a run-in with Sally (Jane Fonda). Thorazine is used to calm Luke (Jon Voight) when he is aggressively swinging a cane and yelling at the healthcare workers about the poor care he gets. These movies are focused on the consequences of the Vietnam War and suggest deplorable healthcare in VA hospitals and are less about care of the paraplegic.

Quotable Lines of Dialogue

Coming Home	
Luke to Sally	*People look at me, but they see something else; and they do not see who I am. Do you know when I dream, I dream I do not have a chair in my dream?*

Another notable film is *The Waterdance* (1992) ⁀⁀ by the paraplegic director Neal Jimenez. The film is virtually fully set in a VA hospital for spine injury and shows the anger and frustration of going through the rehabilitation process. The title is based on a dream of one of the paraplegics where he imagines he has to dance on water or otherwise will drown. The film is largely focused on prolonged rehabilitation but also focuses on the loss of sexuality and the struggles with that adjustment. The screenwriter here is fascinated by sexuality in the paraplegic. The screenplay often strongly leans toward vulgarity.

But it is not all Hollywood, as a comparable theme, sex and paralysis, is seen in Lars von Trier's *Breaking the Waves* (1996) ✷. In this film, Jan (Stellan Skarsgard) is quadriplegic resulting from an accident on a rig. The film accurately shows the secondary complications of acute spinal cord injury and has graphic scenes of a craniotomy and cervical stabilization. The film is, however, not so much about the injury, and has other complex themes (being good, sacrifice, and faith). The recovery is miraculous and essential to the story.

A Final Word

The films scrutinized here provide a good representation of the emotional duress of paraplegics, but some films use the isolation and major handicap of a paraplegic as a device to—objectionably—evoke pity and devastation. Many disabled people are poor, and undoubtedly wars have increased traumatic paraplegia. Is quality of life after a paralysis all a matter of support and access to care? I cannot tell, but cinema has placed a great emphasis on the major societal issues in patients with acute spinal cord injury.

Further Reading

Bryce TN, Biering-Sorensen F, Finnerup NB, et al. International spinal cord injury pain classification: Part I. Background and description. *Spinal Cord* 2012;50:413–17.

Devivo MJ Epidemiology of traumatic spinal cord injury: trends and future implications. *Spinal Cord* 2012;50:365–72.

Hess MJ, Hough S. Impact of spinal cord injury on sexuality: Broad-based clinical practice intervention and practical application. *J Spinal Cord Med* 2012;35:211–18.

Mayo Clinic. *Guide to living with a spinal cord injury*. New York: Demos Health, 2009.

Selzer ME. *Spinal cord injury*. Sydney, Australia: ReadHowYouWant, 2012.

POLIOMYELITIS IN FILM

Sister Kenny (1946); starring Rosalind Russell, Alexander Knox, Philip Merivale, and John Litel; directed by Dudley Nichols, screenplay by Dudley Nichols, Alexander Knox, and Mary McCarthy; Golden Globe Award for best actress; distributed by RKO Radio Pictures.

Rating

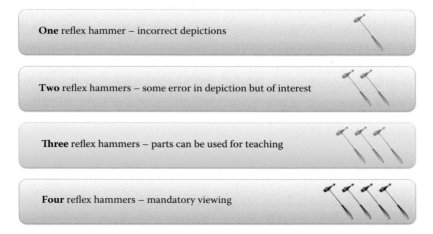

The Sessions (2012); starring John Hawkes, Helen Hunt, and William Macy; written and directed by Ben Lewin; Special Jury Prize for ensemble acting at the 2012 Sundance Film Festival, and John Hawkes and Helen Hunt received the Independent Spirit Award for best male lead and best supporting female; distributed by Fox Searchlight Pictures.

Rating

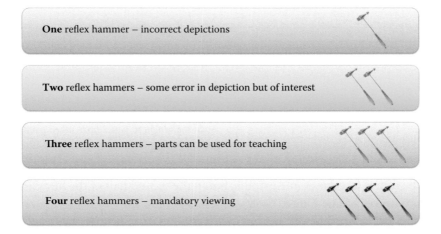

Criticism and Context

Although poliomyelitis is very rare today and most neurologists see the sequelae after many decades have past, this was not the case in the beginning of the twentieth century. Here we discuss two key films, separated by half a century.

An impressive but overly dramatized biopic is *Sister Kenny*, directed by Dudley Nichols and played by Oscar-nominated Rosalind Russell. The film shows her taking the nurse's oath—"With loyalty will I endeavor to aid the physician in his work." (At the time the term sister had been used to indicate nurse, but in reality Sister Kenny had no formal nursing training.) Several confrontational scenes occur in the movie; for example, when Sister Kenny questions the orthopedic surgeon, Dr. Brack (Philip Merivale), regarding his treatment. According to Dr. Brack, "The only thing that offers any hope is prompt and complete immobilization" and "Stick to nursing and don't meddle with orthopedic medicine." The movie suggests that all cases treated by Sister Kenny recovered, that the overwhelming majority treated by orthopedic surgeons were crippled, and that most orthopedic surgeons wanted nothing to do with her methods. The film is more about a major nurse–physician conflict than about Kenny's treatment methods and efficacy (or lack thereof). In this film, it is clearly suggested that patients would get cured if only her methods were used and if only physicians were more accepting and not so arrogant.

Quotable Lines of Dialogue

Sister Kenny	
Kenny to Dr. Brack	*I do not think you are ignorant, only pigheaded. I get improvements even with your failures.*
Kenny to Dr. Brack	*If you need any more braces, steel corsets, or other instruments of medieval torture, I can send them to you. I have taken plenty off your patients.*

The film is largely set in Australia, but in the second half of the film Sister Kenny moves to the United States, where she feels she is getting the runaround and is brushed off. In the final scene she demonstrates her method to orthopedic surgeons, but the film ends not that well when she is told that a US committee also does not support her methods. The film ends with her sitting defeated in a chair. She lights up when children (recovered patients) sing happy birthday to her. (Reportedly, Sister Kenny did not like the ending of the film and it is easy to see why.)

So what really happened with Sister Kenny? Although poliomyelitis is a neurologic disease, it became orthopedic surgeons' territory during the fin de siècle. Restoration of function and transplantation of tendons was commonplace, and that explains their interest. Neurologists would see patients often to confirm the diagnosis but actual care was with rehabilitation physicians, and, when severe respiratory failure occurred, with anesthesiologists. Care seems to have been established until Sister Kenny appeared.

Elizabeth Kenny (Figure 3.6), has been accused of showing fanciful optimism. She came to the United States in 1940 and wrote a major text, *And They Shall Walk*, in 1943. A Queensland commission concluded that the management of wrapping stiffened limbs in hot woolen sheets and "re-educating" the underused muscles by exercising and avoidance of orthopedic splints was no more beneficial than orthodox treatment. Physicians hypothesized that paralyzed muscles could be affected by stretch and that it could reduce deformities. Massage was avoided due to extreme tenderness, but also the use of splints (steel frames) and plaster casts, even if needed to keep the legs in good position. Treatment involved warmth and heat lamps. Therapy for polio was mostly hydrotherapy, massage, and controlled exercises. Electrotherapy was popular in France, but nothing was proven.

The five principles of Kenny's treatment were maintenance of a bright mental outlook, maintenance of "impulse," hydrotherapy (including alternating hot and cold douches), maintenance of circulation, and avoidance of generally accepted methods of immobilization. She did not believe polio affected the nerves but pointed to the muscles that were in spasm and this could be relieved with hot packs and hot blankets. (What she meant by these "spasms," however, remained unresolved, and when a dozen patients and over 3,000 muscle groups were examined by neurologists, none of these "spasms" were found.)

The treatment, with all its controversies, became politicized, in particular after the 1952 epidemic a decade later. Kenny established the Sister Kenny Institute in Minneapolis (now Courage Kenny Rehabilitation Institute) after it appeared that her method remarkably improved outcome in polio patients. Kenny said, when questioned, "Let my record speak." She wrote a book in 1943 with the supportive orthopedic surgeon J.F. Pohl, *The Kenny Concept of Infantile Paralysis and its Treatment*.

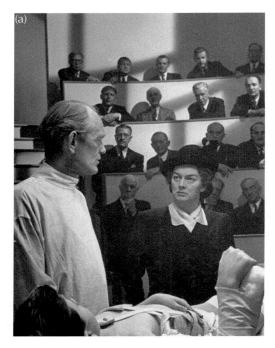

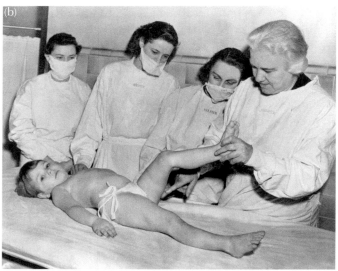

FIGURE 3.6 (a) Scene from *Sister Kenny* showing a confrontational scene with Dr. Brack over a patient's treatment. (Used with permission of Getty Images.) (b) Elisabeth (Sister) Kenny. (Used with permission of Minnesota Historical Society.)

Although Sister Kenny could be abrasive, there are several personal accounts (according to neurologist Donald Mulder, "Sister Kenny was a feisty person who, one observer noted, would continue to fight long after one agreed with her"). There are other accounts that she had moments when she was down in the dumps and she was finding it hard to cope with the large waves of negative publicity. No question Sister Kenny improved care with early mobilization, possibly avoiding unnecessary reconstructive surgeries and a generally far more optimistic approach. Kenny's emphasis on alienation of a paralyzed limb is a real phenomenon and the phenomenon is not only seen in polio but in any long-term immobilized limb.

The Sessions is directed by a childhood polio survivor and is based on a true story. Mark O'Brien died in 1999 after being confined to an iron lung following childhood poliomyelitis. He recalls getting weak and coming out of a coma while encased in an iron lung. (Bulbar poliomyelitis often involves the ascending reticular formation and may lead to coma from hypercapnia.) His parents were told the life expectancy of polio survivors was poor. ("They took me home and gave me a life—gave up theirs.") He was the topic of an Oscar-winning short documentary by Jessica Yu in 1996, *Breathing Lessons: The Life and Work of Mark O'Brien.* (The documentary is a necessary supplement to this film and demands viewing.) Mark O'Brien attended the UC Berkeley Graduate School of Journalism in Berkeley, California, and became a poet and journalist. In 1997, he co-founded Lemonade Factory, a press that publishes work by people who have disabilities. His books include the memoir *How I Became a Human Being: A Disabled Man's Quest for Independence* (2003) and the poetry collections *The Man in the Iron Lung* (1997) and *Breathing* (1998). *Sessions* is structured around an article he wrote, "On Seeing a Sex Surrogate," and handles the topic of sex and disability discreetly.

The film shows the devastating effects of living in an iron lung (he was able to get out of the device for about 3–4 hours per day and slept in it) and living supine for most of the time. He is able to use a portable respirator that allows him to go outside. Respiratory involvement usually affected 10% of the cases, but in some instances it involved up to one-third of the afflicted adults. Patients with severe poliomyelitis often develop sleep apnea, with breathing stopping at the onset of sleep; and in some, the automatic respiratory control during wakefulness may disappear.

John Hawkes plays Mark O'Brien and imitates his voice using short sentences, but not the staccato speech so typical of neuromuscular respiratory failure (catching a breath in between a few words). His body is appropriately skinny (patients may weigh no more than 60 kilograms), and he appropriately imitates the often-seen severe spinal deformities, such as kyphoscoliosis, that often worsen the respiratory problems over time. The movie also shows the severe pain with movements of limbs in severe contracture.

Quotable Lines of Dialogue

The Sessions	
Mark O'Brien	*This most excellent canopy, the air, look you,*
	Presses down upon me
	At fifteen pounds per square inch,
	A dense, heavy, blue-glowing ocean,
	Supporting the weight of condors
	That swim its churning currents.
	All I get is a thin stream of it,
	A finger's width of the rope that ties me to life
	As I labor like a stevedore to keep the
	connection.
	(Start of the film and excerpted from a poem by Mark O'Brien)

Poliomyelitis has appeared in several screenplays in the past but has disappeared with the near-disappearance of the disorder. One of the first films to deal with the burdens of poliomyelitis is the cold-blooded noir *Leave Her to Heaven* (1945) ⌇⌇, about Ellen (Gene Tierney) and Richard Harland (Cornel Wilde). Ellen and Richard are newlyweds, and Richard's brother Danny (Darryl Hickman) is recovering from poliomyelitis in the well-known rehabilitation center, the Warm Springs Foundation in Georgia. Danny is a Hollywood feel-good example of a happy-go-lucky (see what I can do with crutches!) optimist who can soon leave the rehabilitation center. Ellen is glad to comply with his care, but after his physician suggests to her that he can return home, she gets visibly upset with the idea of having to take him home ("after all, he is a cripple"). His presence puts a wedge in the relationship of the married couple.

He seems to recover and is able to move his legs and do swimming exercises. The film is a thriller, and the femme fatale Ellen watches him drown in an iconic scene, where she fakes a rescue attempt after he has drowned. Interestingly, nowhere in the script is poliomyelitis specifically mentioned; it is only implied.

Polio is used to great effect in *The Five Pennies* (1959). ᐟ Danny Kaye plays the band leader, and at the end of the film his daughter is affected. We see her in a few scenes in an iron long, recovering in a hospital bed through rehabilitation to eventually walking with a cane and dancing again with her father. The director knew what the audience wanted to see—full recovery of poliomyelitis against all odds and physician prediction. (This clinical course is not very likely.) It also shows Sister Kenny's hot compresses and Danny Kaye goofing off to try to raise his daughter's spirits. He puts blankets on her legs ("the most delicious thing your mother cooked since we're in this house…blanket a la mode"), buys her a puppy, and so forth, but the film is not about poliomyelitis.

What can be said about poliomyelitis to better understand the portrayal? Poliomyelitis is a viral infection by an enterovirus that in the overwhelming proportion of cases causes a nondistinctive viral illness, and in some a devastating paralysis from involvement of the anterior horn of the spinal cord. When the brainstem becomes involved, patients have difficulty clearing secretions from oropharyngeal weakness, and respiration becomes compromised. Many of these patients in the past had back stiffness and severe pain from hypertonicity. Many patients developed intercostal paralysis and severe weakness of the diaphragm, an early paralytic stage of anterior poliomyelitis. In many, the accessory muscles and the diaphragm were able to create sufficient respiratory movements. In the course of a few days, the paralyzed intercostal muscles improved, and the patient went on to almost complete recovery.

Respiratory support involved the infamous "iron lung." This machine incorporated electrically driven blowers and created inspiration with negative pressures and expiration with positive pressure (Figure 3.7). Within the chamber—sealing the patient at the neck—a negative pressure caused the abdomen and thorax to expand with air flowing in. A cycle is produced by returning to atmospheric pressure. Patients in the iron lung have their chest expanded every 4 seconds. Many patients have been able to be liberated from the device or transitioned to a cuirass ventilator. During the major epidemics the iron lung was seen as a temporary lifesaving machine, but later it became clear that weaning was not possible and respiratory support would now have a permanent impact on the quality of the patient's existence (Chapter 5).

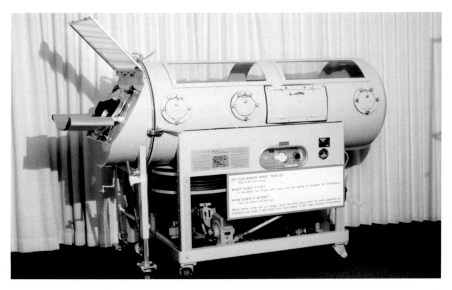

FIGURE 3.7 Iron lung. (Used with permission of Mayo Historical Unit and Archives.)

A Final Word

Film deals with poliomyelitis in different ways—the burden of "a cripple," the arrogant orthopedic surgeons not accepting a nursing approach, a life in an iron lung, and in general living with a paralyzed body. The spectrum covered cannot be more all-encompassing and is of more than just historical interest. It acknowledges the importance that poliomyelitis epidemics played in people's lives, in medical history, and in the history of critical care medicine. Poliomyelitis still has not been eradicated. (For further discussion on poliomyelitis, see Chapter 5.)

Further Reading

Commission RoQ. Treatment of infantile paralysis by Sister Kenny's method. *Br Med J (Clin Res Ed)* 1938;1:350.

Drinker P, McKhann CF. The use of a new apparatus for the prolonged administration of artificial respiration: I. A fatal case of poliomyelitis. *JAMA* 1929;92:1658–60.

Kendall FP. Sister Elizabeth Kenny revisited. *Arch Phys Med Rehabil* 1998;79:361–65.

Oshinsky DM. *Polio: An American story*. 2nd ed. New York: Oxford University Press, 2006.

Rogers N. *Polio wars: Sister Kenny and the golden age of American medicine*. New York: Oxford University Press, 2013.

MULTIPLE SCLEROSIS IN FILM

Go Now (1995); starring Robert Carlyle, Juliet Aubrey, and James Nesbitt; directed by Michael Winterbottom, written by Jimmy McGovern and Paul Henry Powell; BAFTA Award for best editing; distributed by Gramercy Pictures.

Rating

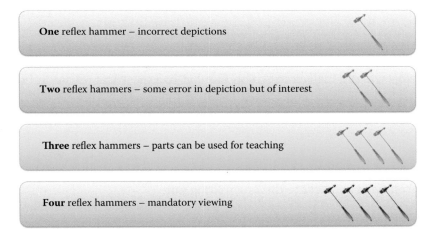

One reflex hammer – incorrect depictions

Two reflex hammers – some error in depiction but of interest

Three reflex hammers – parts can be used for teaching

Four reflex hammers – mandatory viewing

Hilary and Jackie (1998); starring Emily Watson, Rachel Griffiths, James Frain, and David Morrissey; directed by Anand Tucker, written by Frank Cottrell Boyce; Academy Award for best actress (Emily Watson) and for best supporting actress (Rachel Griffith), BAFTA Award for best British film; distributed by Channel 4 Films.

Rating

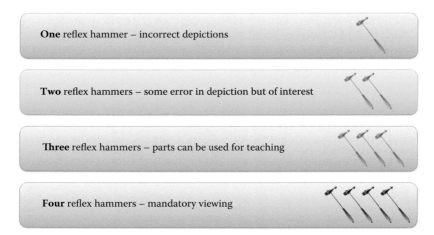

One reflex hammer – incorrect depictions

Two reflex hammers – some error in depiction but of interest

Three reflex hammers – parts can be used for teaching

Four reflex hammers – mandatory viewing

Criticism and Context

Two major films, both by UK directors (Michael Winterbottom and Anand Tucker), have placed multiple sclerosis (MS) prominently in their films. *Go Now* was originally a television film but had theatrical release in both the United Kingdom and United States. It follows Nick (Robert Carlyle) and Karen (Juliet Aubrey) and their struggle with progressive MS. Nick, a working-class Glaswegian, develops a useless hand followed by numbness, ataxic-spastic gait, and eventually double vision. The ophthalmologist refuses to tell the diagnosis, afraid it will lead to more stress. The neurologist procrastinates and adds to the long waiting time.

Quotable Lines of Dialogue

Go Now	
Karen	*All those questions you are asking him. He has got MS?*
Ophthalmologist	*Not necessarily. It is a possibility.*
Karen	*Why the hell did you not tell him?*
Ophthalmologist	*Do you know anything about MS?*
Karen	*A bit.*
Ophthalmologist	*The symptoms can come and go. Sometimes they disappear altogether.*
Karen	*If he's got it, he has the right to know.*
Ophthalmologist	*It is stress related. Telling him might induce an attack.*
Karen	*What are you going to do?*
Ophthalmologist	*Nothing; but if you want to tell him, you should do so.*

Go Now is a film that shines light on the frustrations of diagnosis of MS and coping with the handicap. The film plays in a time where the diagnosis was more difficult to make due to lack of wide availability of magnetic resonance (MR) imaging and perhaps also due to cautious physicians who would not commit to definitive conclusions.

The first sign of Nick's MS is numbness, resulting in a sledgehammer falling down a shaft. Soon he has blurred vision, leading to an extensive ophthalmologic evaluation with visual field testing. "You won't make the dart team," his girlfriend Karen (Juliet Aubrey) jokingly remarks. The ophthalmologist calls it a "trapped nerve and overcompensating," resulting in a new eyeglass prescription. These symptoms worry Karen, and she goes to the library and finds out that these signs could mean MS. Another meeting follows, and the film shows a conversation with the ophthalmologist, where he suggests withholding the diagnosis. Such reluctance has been predicated on the uncertainty of predicting the course of MS. The scene reflects what might have been the practice in the United Kingdom (and elsewhere in the 1960s) but not in current office practices. Neurologists tell patients the diagnosis when there is a reasonable certainty of MS and on the basis of actual evidence.

In the ensuing scenes, Nick has great difficulty to move his foot and is unable to stop his car from crashing. Next he is walking in the hospital with a spastic gait but without any information. ("There is something wrong with me. They are testing for AIDS.") He leaves the hospital, and much to his surprise, discovers that his girlfriend has an MS self-help book. This leads to a confrontation and finally acceptance. Nick's MS progresses with incontinence and impotence but has a "happy ending" while they are dancing at their wedding to the Moody Blues' song, "Go Now." The film has some banalities, but there are many good reasons to see it. The themes chosen in this film are creditable.

Another important film, *Hilary and Jackie*, is based on the late Jacqueline du Pré, her family, and her relationship with her sister. (The film is closely based on Piers and Hilary du Pré's memoir entitled *A Genius in the Family*.) Jacqueline du Pré married Daniel Barenboim, and both became prominent musicians. It was one of the first films dealing with how a progressive neurologic disease could impact a musician's career (see also the section on Parkinson's disease). The film is mostly about the two sisters' close relationship, and her diagnosis of MS does not emerge until 90 minutes into the film. No discussion with a physician is seen. Complaining of cold hands is one of the first premonitory signs presented here, but there is otherwise an accurate portrayal of rapid, progressive MS. Jackie (Emily Watson) starts with having a bow fall out of her hand followed by tremor, incontinence, and an inability to get out of a chair after performing a concert; then her hearing disappears, canes appear, she cannot roll over in bed, and she ends up in a wheelchair. This all plays out in the last 20 minutes of the film, likely to achieve grand effect. Most prominently displayed by Jackie are her emotional mood swings and her euphoric outlook. These affective states are well known in MS, even since Charcot's original description. Uncontrollable laughing and crying, however, is not shown. Jackie is a happy-go-lucky person, although that is often not indicative of the true mood she is in. The film shows spastic ataxia and dystonic (tremor) posturing, all consistent with primary progressive MS. In the early stages, there is a brief mention of "pills" to allow her to play her instrument, but no specific treatment is mentioned.

Quotable Lines of Dialogue

Hilary and Jackie	
Jackie	*I have got a fatal illness, but you must not worry. I got it very mildly.*
Jackie	*I am so relieved it is only MS. I know it is serious, but I thought I was going mad.*

Hilary and Jackie is based on medical reports and witness reports. A recent study of MS portrayal in the movies by Karenberg concluded adequate portrayal, but this review also included horror and TV movies. Visual symptoms are underrepresented. Sensational contextualization was absent in most films. A very different and strange film is *Dreamland* (2006), which shows a young woman with MS and "killer spasms." She uses bee stings and she touches electrical wires to improve her condition. The films that use MS in their plots, unfortunately, use it to show a major disabling disease ending in major handicap and ignore the much more common unpredictable and benign nature. Treatments are rarely mentioned, if ever.

A Final Word

The worldwide prevalence of MS is approximately 2 million individuals. Many patients are asymptomatic. A third of patients will be without major symptoms at 10 years and 20% at 20 years. It is likely that progression of MS nowadays is influenced by new therapeutic approaches in the acute and chronic phases. Both *Go Now* and *Hilary and Jackie* show a rapid progressive—likely primary progressive—MS (see documentary in Chapter 5). Both films may lead to public misconceptions that MS rapidly leads to use of a wheelchair and fatality.

Further Reading

Confavreux C, Vukusic S. Age at disability milestones in multiple sclerosis. *Brain* 2006;129:595–605.

Corona T, Poser C, Du Pré J. Talent and disease. *Neurologia* 2004;19:85.

Finger S. A happy state of mind: A history of mild elation, denial of disability, optimism, and laughing in multiple sclerosis. *Arch Neurol* 1998;55:241–50.

Kalincik T, Vivek V, Jokubaitis V, et al. Sex as a determinant of relapse incidence and progressive course of multiple sclerosis. *Brain* 2013;12:3609–17.

Karenberg A. Multiple sclerosis on-screen: From disaster to coping. *Mult Scler* 2008;14:530–40.

Weiner HL, Stankiewicz JM, eds. *Multiple sclerosis: Diagnosis and therapy*. 2nd ed. New York: Wiley-Blackwell, 2012.

MOTOR NEURON DISEASE IN FILM

Tuesdays with Morrie (1999); starring Jack Lemmon and Hank Azaria; directed by Mick Jackson, written by Thomas Rickman, based on a novel by Mitch Albom; distributed by Carlton America, Harpo Productions.

Rating

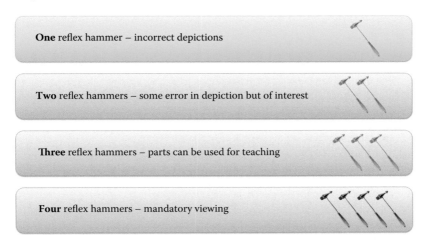

One reflex hammer – incorrect depictions

Two reflex hammers – some error in depiction but of interest

Three reflex hammers – parts can be used for teaching

Four reflex hammers – mandatory viewing

The Theory of Flight (1998); Helena Bonham Carter, Kenneth Branagh, and Gemma Jones; directed by Paul Greengrass, written by Richard Hawkins; distributed by First Line Features.

Rating

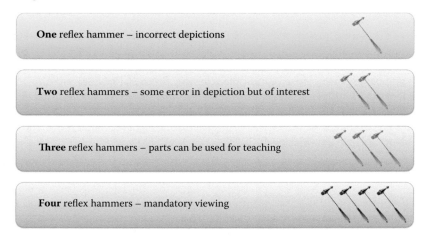

One reflex hammer – incorrect depictions

Two reflex hammers – some error in depiction but of interest

Three reflex hammers – parts can be used for teaching

Four reflex hammers – mandatory viewing

Hugo Pool (1997); starring Alicia Milano, Patrick Dempsey, and Robert Downey Jr.; directed by Robert Downey Sr.; distributed by Northern Arts Entertainment.

Rating

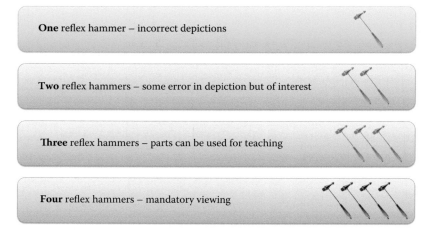

One reflex hammer – incorrect depictions

Two reflex hammers – some error in depiction but of interest

Three reflex hammers – parts can be used for teaching

Four reflex hammers – mandatory viewing

Criticism and Context

Motor neuron disease is not a topic readily chosen by screenwriters, and when it is used, it seems to fall into the general categories of "severe disability" and "dying from an untreatable disorder." There are very few fiction films to consider, and the best-known movie *Tuesdays with Morrie* is based on Mitch Albom's tremendously popular best-selling novel about Morrie Schwartz, who died of amyotrophic lateral sclerosis (ALS). The film is about one of Morrie's students, Mitch Albom, who travels every week from Detroit to Boston to meet with him. The film's main theme is for Mitch to come to the realization that a fatal illness can be unnecessarily prolonged.

Morrie decides that he will not proceed with a tracheostomy and mechanical ventilation when he reaches the inevitable progression to severe swallowing difficulties. The film is about acceptance. ("Don't treat me. I'm already dead.") It is about what matters in life more than about the disorder of ALS. In Albom's book, it is clear that Morrie never spoke about his illness or his own coping with becoming disabled. The film shows the young seeing the life experiences of the old and dying. Both the film and the book may be characterized by some as a touchy-feely story about the gradual decline of a virtuous man and "love conquers all," but does not provide insight into the specific tortuous decline of ALS. Overall, the main criticisms of the book involved its simplicity, and that also applies to this movie.

Two other films have specifically used motor neuron disease (and ALS), and both actors seem to be modeled after Stephen Hawking, the British physicist diagnosed with motor neuron disease at the age of 21 (he is now 71 years old). His diagnosis, a variant of ALS, may better fit with a progressive muscular atrophy or primary lateral sclerosis. His posture, with a lateral head deviation, is used by both actors. In *The Theory of Flight* (1998), Jane (Helena Bonham Carter) is a disabled woman with a "rare form of motor neuron disease." The film is mostly about how she can lose her virginity. She communicates with a voice box and seems to closely imitate Stephen Hawking's appearance. She lifts one of her shoulders to her head, creating a similar look, and speaks with poor articulation and lack of mimicry.

In *Hugo Pool*, Patrick Dempsey plays Floyd. He is in a wheelchair and also has a voice box. In the film, it becomes clear that he wants everyone to know that ALS is not contagious and that his lovemaking is not fully affected.

Quotable Lines of Dialogue

Hugo Pool	
Minerva	*My daughter says you got this thing, ALS. What does it do to you?*
	It attacks the nerves and then they die.
	The only part that does not get destroyed is the brain.
Floyd	*I got a twitch in my right arm. That is what happens before*
	I lose it.
Hugo	*You are going to beat it.*
Floyd	*I like the way you think.*

His role is central in the movie—in a wheelchair, not moving, not speaking (only a whisper), being spoon-fed and drinking through a straw. His head is constantly tilted to one side, also likely mimicking Stephen Hawking's posture. Predictably, in one of the final scenes he has sexual intercourse with Hugo (Alyssa Milano) and soon thereafter passes away.

Both films have little to say about motor neuron disease and are about living with a major disability and—how can it not be in classic entertainment—about sex in a markedly disabled person.

A Final Word

All three films represent ALS poorly—in an end stage but with major inconsistencies, unable to speak but still able to safely eat. There are no redeeming qualities in any of these films. Serious viewers should turn to the documentaries (discussed in Chapter 5), which are a stunning antidote to the ridiculousness of these portrayals.

Further Reading

Belsh JM. Diagnostic challenges in ALS. *Neurology* 1999;53:S26–30; discussion S35–36.

Francis K, Bach JR, DeLisa JA. Evaluation and rehabilitation of patients with adult motor neuron disease. *Arch Phys Med Rehabil* 1999;80:951–63.

Gordon PH, Cheng B, Katz IB, Mitsumoto H, Rowland LP. Clinical features that distinguish PLS, upper motor neuron-dominant ALS, and typical ALS. *Neurology* 2009;72:1948–52.

Winter RO, Birnberg BA. Tuesdays with Morrie versus Stephen Hawking: Living or dying with ALS. *Fam Med* 2003;35:629–31.

LEPROSY IN FILM

The Motorcycle Diaries (2004); starring Gael Garcia Bernal and Rodrigo de la Serna; directed by Walter Salles, written by Jose Rivera; BAFTA Award for best film not in English language, among other awards; distributed by Focus Features.

Rating

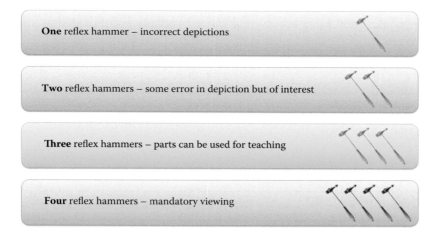

One reflex hammer – incorrect depictions

Two reflex hammers – some error in depiction but of interest

Three reflex hammers – parts can be used for teaching

Four reflex hammers – mandatory viewing

Criticism and Context

The Motorcycle Diaries is based on a memoir of Ernesto Guevara, who went on a journey from Argentina through Chile, Peru, Colombia, and Venezuela, which included the San Pablo leper colony. The leper colony is a key element in the film. His friend Alberto Granado, who had already worked in a leprosy hospital in Cordoba, Argentina, was the one who initiated the trip. Ernesto Guevara de la Serna (later known as Che Guevara) was an Argentine medical student who dropped out of medical school to join Alberto on this defining trip. The film has little to say about his later political activism. Here it concentrates on his confrontation with the leprosarium, where approximately 600, mostly Peruvian, patients were under the care of missionaries.

The island is separated by the Amazon river (the medical staff lives on the other side of the river). When Ernesto crosses the river, a physician asks him to wear gloves, but he refuses, and when he visits the colony, he shakes hands, to the surprise of a patient. ("Doctor, haven't you explained the rules?") Most of the patients with leprosy live there after having been fired from their jobs, and now they raise farm animals. The film shows real patients affected by leprosy, their major mutilations and nodular skin lesions resulting from granulomatous disease. In the three weeks that Ernesto and Alberto stay in this leprosarium, they attend to wound care and convince Sylvia ("a rebellious patient") to proceed with surgery to save her arm. The visit ends with a historically accurate farewell scene by Ernesto when he swims across the Amazon River. The film correctly depicts the concentration of leprosy in leprosariums, often on islands. These leprosariums stigmatized patients but provided accurate management of the disease, often under the guidance of missionaries.

Quotable Lines of Dialogue

The Motorcycle Diaries	
Doctor	*I suggest you wear these gloves although leprosy is not contagious under treatment. The nuns are quite insistent on this point.*
Ernesto	*If it's not contagious, then it is just symbolic.*
Doctor	*Yes, but I'm telling you so you don't make any mortal enemies. Don't say I did not warn you.*

Leprosy is a granulomatous infection of both nerves and skin caused by *Mycobacterium leprae*. It is still a significant health problem, and the World Health Assembly continues with measures to eliminate leprosy throughout the world. A significant improvement occurred after initiation of multidrug therapy following many centuries of dapsone treatment. Leprosy is typically diagnosed as hypopigmented or reddish patches with loss of sensation, markedly thickened peripheral nerves, followed by nerve injury and weakness and documentation of acid-fast bacilli on skin smears or biopsy material. Nerve damage involves the peripheral nerve trunks and more specifically on a radial cutaneous nerve, medial nerve, postural tibial nerve, and the lateral popliteal nerve. Enlargement of these nerves may cause pain but eventually also produces hypesthesia and hyperhidrosis, which results in infections and ulceration. Treatment is rifampicin, clofazimine, and dapsone. There is uncertainty about transmission, and it has been known for many years that proximity to leprosy patients increases the risk. However, bacteria do not enter intact skin and they are not spread through touch.

The film clearly identifies the presence of missionaries and their role in treating leprosy. In the beginning of the last century, there were thousands of European missionaries serving in many parts of the country with their objective not only to serve lepers, but also to engage in evangelization. Often the biblical base of their mission was based on New Testament passages that include miracles performed on lepers who came to Jesus asking for cleansing and casting out demons. This is also clearly reflected in *The Motorcycle Diaries*, when Mother Superior refuses food to Ernesto and Alberto because they did not attend Holy Mass. However, the importance of missionary work in treatment of those affected by leprosy cannot be overstated.

City of Joy (1992) ⨞, with Patrick Swayze, shows slums in Calcutta, India, with actual patients with leprosy, and the noninfectious origin is again emphasized. ("I have it, but my daughter does not.") There is one remarkable line by one of the doctors saying that these people are simple and not educated, and they will never accept lepers in their midst. (City of Joy Aid is actually a humanitarian organization in Calcutta, and the network of clinics, schools, rehabilitation centers, and hospital boats bring relief to the most needy.)

In *The Hawaiians* (1970), there is a very brief scene showing crippled lepers separated on an island who are pushed away by the lead actor (Charlton Heston) in the film, but without much further insight into the disorder. The lepers look like zombies.

A Final Word

Leprosy is a major neurologic disease and has been mentioned in several films. *The Motorcycle Diaries*, where an actual leper colony is used, is the best example.

Leprosy is not eradicated outside the Western world, with a prevalence of more than 1 per 10,000 in Asia, Africa, and South America. The World Health Organization has found major concentrations of leprosy in India, Brazil, Burma, Madagascar, and Nepal. There has been an increase over the last decade, possibly explained by improved case finding.

Further Reading

Britton WJ, Lockwood DN. Leprosy. *Lancet* 2004;363:1209–19.
Foss NT, Motta AC. Leprosy, a neglected disease that causes a wide variety of clinical conditions in tropical countries. *Mem Inst Oswaldo Cruz* 2012;107 Suppl 1:28–33.

Kipp RS. The evangelical uses of leprosy. *Soc Sci Med* 1994;39:165–78.

Rodrigues LC, Lockwood D. Leprosy now: Epidemiology, progress, challenges, and research gaps. *Lancet Infect Dis* 2011;11:464–70.

Williams DL, Gillis TP. Drug-resistant leprosy: Monitoring and current status. *Lepr Rev* 2012;83:269–81.

World Health Organization. Global strategy for further reducing the leprosy burden and sustaining leprosy control activities (2006–2010): Operational guidelines. 2006. http://www1.paho.org/English/AD/DPC/CD/lep-global-strat-06-op-gl.htm (accessed April 8, 2014).

AMNESIA IN FILM

Memento (2000); starring Guy Pearce, Carrie-Anne Moss, and Joe Pantoliano; directed by Christopher Nolan; distributed by Summit Entertainment.

Rating

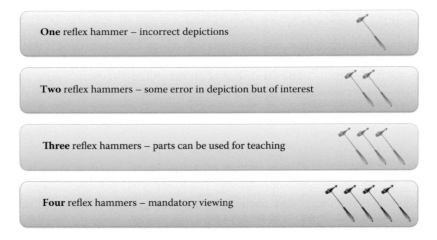

One reflex hammer – incorrect depictions

Two reflex hammers – some error in depiction but of interest

Three reflex hammers – parts can be used for teaching

Four reflex hammers – mandatory viewing

The Music Never Stopped (2011); starring Lou Taylor Pucci, J.K. Simmons, and Julia Ormond; directed by Jim Kohlberg, written by Gwyn Lurie and Gary Marks; distributed by Essential Pictures.

Rating

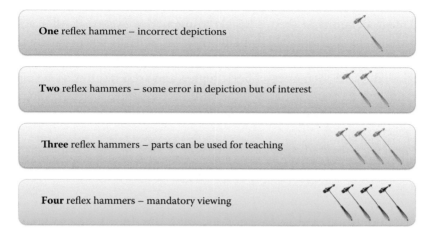

The Vow (2012); starring Rachel McAdams, Channing Tatum, Sam Neill, and Jessica Lange; directed by Michael Sucsy, written by Abby Kohn, Marc Silverstein, and Jason Katims; distributed by Screen Gems.

Rating

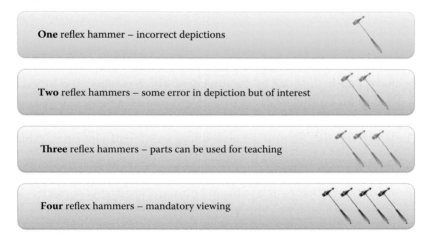

Criticism and Context

Memory difficulties have attracted screenwriters, and one can immediately imagine why: Wouldn't it be entertaining if the leading character cannot remember what he or she has done? Many films have used this plot device, but three films stand out.

Antegrade amnesia (being unable to memorize events) is often used. This should be differentiated from dissociative amnesia, where patients are aware they have lost their memories. Unplanned travel and unknown personal identity are seen in psychiatric fugues and are a result of a traumatic stressful event. Such travel is often also accompanied by psychological inability to recall the past. (Travis, in *Paris, Texas* [1984] by Wim Wenders, is a good example.)

Memento is focused on Lenny Shelby (Guy Pierce). Lenny has lost all ability to remember. "I can't make new memories. Everything just fades." The film is told in reverse order, is fragmented, and reflects the true condition. The film is also very dense, and many fans of this film who have scrutinized and combed through the scenes multiple times are still asking questions.

Quotable Lines of Dialogue

Memento

Leonard

I have to believe in a world outside my own mind. I have to believe that my actions still have meaning, even if I can't remember them. I have to believe that when my eyes are closed, the world's still there. Do I believe the world's still there? Is it still out there? Yeah. We all need mirrors to remind ourselves who we are. I am no different.

In short, Lenny kills one of the intruders who has raped and killed his wife. He gets hit on the head, causing anterograde amnesia. Lenny makes Polaroids of places and written notes. His body has tattoos with clues to the killer of his wife. The movie also shows a different plot line (in black and white), where Leonard is introduced as an insurance investigator. He is investigating a man with anterograde amnesia but is accused of "faking it." Proof of that is that he is unable to be conditioned. It is correctly posited here that, although he cannot make memories, he still should be able to develop conditioning for situations that could harm him. In order to see if he is "faking it," his wife tries an experiment and asks him to give her insulin injections (which he does all the time). She secretly turns back the clock in the room so it seems no time has passed, asks it again and again until she becomes comatose (and never recovers). The film's dramatic proof that his condition is real and not fake is essentially correct, and in reality this type of situation could theoretically happen in persons with such memory loss.

The Music Never Stopped is based on an actual patient reported by Oliver Sacks in his essay "The Last Hippie" from his book *An Anthropologist on Mars: Seven Paradoxical Tales* (1995). The patient described by neurologist Oliver Sacks was Gabriel Sawyer, who had a large meningioma extending into the diencephalon that was destroying optic chiasm as well as the frontal and temporal lobes. Gabriel was told by his swami that he was "an illuminate" and was becoming a saint. This interpretation delayed surgery.

After surgery Gabriel had marked difficulty remembering events from the 1960s and nothing after 1970. He could play the guitar but he was unable to generate any immediate memories. He displayed frontal syndrome in the form of "wisecracking." There was also increased word play. ("Lunch is here, it is time to cheer.") He tried to learn Braille but was unable to and could not grasp the reason for it. ("Why am I here with blind people?")

Oliver Sacks met one of the Grateful Dead band members and took Gabriel to a concert (who did light up and said he "had the time of my life"), but he did forget about it the next day. According to Sacks, Gabriel recognized all the songs but not those written after 1970; he recognized the style, though, thinking that it could be something the Grateful Dead might write some day. The film shows him in the hospital with an advanced brain tumor and loss of sight. The parents' conversation with the neurosurgeon, which is notable and comical, and he explains that the tumor is benign, but that he may be left with a major deficit after surgery. (The neurosurgeon [played by Scott Adsit]) points to the thalamus and incorrectly calls it the forebrain. When Gabriel's father asks, "So the tumor is in this area?" the neurosurgeon responds, irritated, "No, Mr. Sawyer, that is the tumor." Next we see the neurosurgeon examining Gabriel after surgery, and he asks him to count from 1 to 10, to which Gabriel answers, "Count me out."

The film shows him in a skilled nursing facility where he plays "La Marseillaise" on trumpet and asks others what song it is. The film then dramatically shows that during music therapy, Gabriel suddenly transforms from a frozen (abulic and catatonic) state to being animated and alive. (According to Oliver Sacks, his patient could not engage in a social conversation, but music elicited strong memories of lyrics and emotions.)

Although he has marked anterograde amnesia, he could remember all the songs of the 1960s and 1970s. When he sees a girl in the cafeteria who is named Cecilia, he sings Simon and Garfunkel's song *Cecilia* ("Oh, Cecilia, you're breaking my heart") every time he sees her.

The movie mostly coalescences into a renewed connection between father and estranged son through the music of the Grateful Dead, Bob Dylan, Crosby, Stills, and Nash, and other rock stars from the "flower power" era. The movie touches on the mystery of music and emotions.

It has been known that songs or musical pieces become encoded or hardwired in the brain and can be retrieved similarly as with familiar faces. Such an experience may be different in a musician, but this oddity of profound amnesia—a catatonic state but "awakening" when favorite songs are heard—is a major interest of Oliver Sacks (see also Chapter 5). The film may prompt a discussion on music and the brain. For many of us, it remains a poorly understood field.

A more recent film that involves an improbable amnesia is *The Vow* (2012). A traumatic head injury leaves Paige (Rachel McAdams) comatose. The film shows her still looking stunning with a few scratches and perfectly coiffed. After her surgery, we are told she is "kept" comatose using sedation. She awakens with a selective memory loss of the past 5 years, and she does not recognize her husband, Leo (Channing Tatum) but does recognize her parents. When she meets her siblings, she recognizes them ("everyone looks older") and also friends from high school. The rest of the plot shows her gradually becoming aware of some prior relationships, but not all of them. There is a notable scene with her neurosurgeon (or neurologist), who looks at pupil reflexes and asks her about her memory and if she wants to regain her memory. The doctor warns Paige that she does not have to be afraid she would remember the accident ("Mercifully, that is rarely the case") and advises her to try to get her memory back. "I only did one psych rotation so this may be terrible advice, but I think you should try to fill the holes."

Two types of amnesia occur after traumatic head injury. Anterograde amnesia is typically impaired new learning and forgetting. Retrograde amnesia is deficits in memory storage or retrieval. Psychogenic amnesia is not restricted to a single event (usually hours before the event), but involves a large part of the past. (It often affects young people.)

This memory deficit may last for years. These patients are unable to recall information before the onset of the event, but anterograde memory is intact. Many may have sudden loss of the ability to read or write or use the telephone.

In a critical review, Baxendale concluded that the movies have the amnesic syndromes wrong. Her major findings are: (1) films do not distinguish between amnesia from a psychiatric illness or underlying neurologic cause; (2) retrograde amnesia exists despite intact capacity for new learning; (3) a second head injury can cure amnesia from a first head injury; (4) memories are temporarily inaccessible, not lost.

Memento is a correct example of amnesia, and the closest resemblance is of a real patient, Henry Molaison (also known as H.M.), who developed anterograde memory impairment after epilepsy surgery. (Although many critics have made a link between the film and his case history, the clinical course for H.M. was not known to the screenwriter, and the film was not inspired by his medical history.)

Henry Molaison (Figure 3.8) was treated for intractable seizures with removal of both medial temporal lobes that included important structures such as the hippocampus (space orientation and backing up of memory) and amygdala (also memory consolidation and human emotions). He was left with permanent amnesia, and his neuropsychologic profile was recently summarized in Suzanne Corkin's book, aptly titled *Permanent Present Tense*. Each time he met someone, it was for the first time. The abundant research found that he could not hold on to thoughts for more than 20 seconds. His motor tasks (things he learned in the past) were intact, so he could do routine things such as cleaning the house or fixing a meal. According to Corkin's work, when asked, "What do you try to remember?" he replied, "Well, that I don't know cause I do not remember what I tried." (His sense of humor remained intact.)

According to Corkin's interpretation, Henry proved for the first time that a discrete medial temporal lobe region converts short-term memories into lasting memories. Distinctions between several forms of memory can now be made. These are *episodic memory* (remembrance of unique events), *semantic memory* (remembering facts), *declarative memory* (learning with awareness), and *procedural memory* (learning without awareness such as motor skills). All were defective in Henry except learning of motor skills. Skills that depended on visual perception and motor abilities could be taught to Henry. He also remembered childhood events.

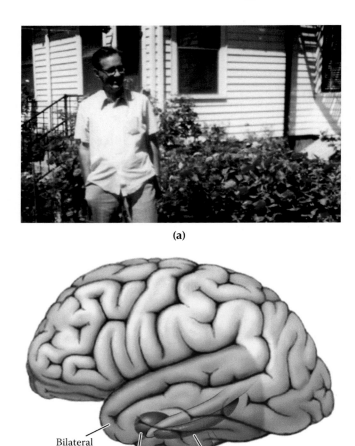

FIGURE 3.8 (a) Henry Molaison. (Used with permission from The Wylie Agency LLC.) (b) The major structures involved with memory are shown in the figure, and the full temporal lobe was removed.

Some other films deserve mention. The Hindi film *Ghajini* (2008) is considered a remake of *Memento* that caused some controversy when Christopher Nolan was not credited. The most extreme form of global amnesia is the movie *Groundhog Day* (1990), where recall of the previous day is absent and is combined with global amnesia of everyone else in the movie. More silliness is apparent in the otherwise tremendously entertaining film *Eternal Sunshine of the Spotless Mind* (2004), where memory is erased with new technology. Another example, *50 First Dates* (2004), is discussed in Chapter 6.

A Final Word

Screenwriters are very interested in loss of memory, but there is little accuracy. Very few films show the frequent presentation of memory difficulties; some things are remembered and others are not. Two key films on amnesia involve dramatic cases—one based on a real patient—and this increases the entertainment value. Understanding memory deficits remains a difficult area for neurologists and neuropsychologists, and very few illuminating cases have been examined.

Further Reading

Bartsch T, Butler C. Transient amnesic syndromes. *Nat Rev Neurol* 2013;9:86–97.
Baxendale S. Memories aren't made of this: Amnesia at the movies. *BMJ* 2004;329:1480–83.
Corkin S. *Permanent present tense: The unforgettable life of the amnesic patient, H.M.* London: Allen Lane, 2013.
Marshman LA, Jakabek D, Hennessy M, Quirk F, Guazzo EP. Post-traumatic amnesia. *J Clin Neurosci* 2013;20:1475–81.

HEADACHE IN FILM

Pi (π) (1998); starring Sean Gullette, Mark Margolis, Ben Shenkman, and Samia Shoaib; written and directed by Darren Aronofsky; distributed by Artisan Entertainment.

Rating

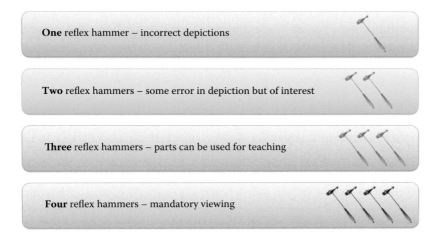

One reflex hammer – incorrect depictions

Two reflex hammers – some error in depiction but of interest

Three reflex hammers – parts can be used for teaching

Four reflex hammers – mandatory viewing

Criticism and Context

As a dramatized depiction, the film *Pi* (π) shows cluster headache well and had an enduring effect on the audience. Although headache does not play any role in advancing the plot, it is part of the struggle of a mathematician to find order in numbers. His assumptions are that mathematics is a language of nature, and that everything can be represented and understood through numbers. If numbers are graphed, certain patterns emerge.

Max Cohen, played by Sean Gullette, often discusses the nature of mathematics with Sol Robeson, played by Mark Margolis. Max is interested in finding a pattern in the stock market but also comes in contact with Lenny Meyer, played by Ben Shenkman. He is interested in the number 216 that represents the letters of the name of God that will open the doors to the Messianic Age. His headaches may be linked to having that number in his head.

The film suggests that his headaches started at the age of 6 years when he was staring at the sun and became "blind." His headaches are repetitive. The film shows, in rapid succession, crosscuts of him popping pills, screeching sounds, hallucinations of moving doors with locks which open up to a bright light. This scene specifically mentions his medications, and he uses promazine and sumatriptan followed by dihydroergotamine mesylate by subcutaneous injection. Multiple attacks are shown, including banging his head against a mirror to relieve the pain and he injects dihydroergotamine into the skin of his skull. Notable here is the large (staple gun–like) injector that must be a deliberate choice by the director to add drama. The film shockingly ends with drilling a burr hole during a severe headache attack.

The film represents cluster headache reasonably well. It shows pain on one side, on the same side as lacrimation, but it does not show ptosis or periorbital edema for an understandable reason. It shows the repetitive nature of the pain. Most patients with cluster headaches have their attacks in the third or fifth decade. The triggers of these headaches are typically wine, nocturnal sleep with daytime naps, and strong odors such as perfume or paint. All of these triggers are shown in this film.

The first treatment of cluster headache is oxygen, but as mentioned in the movie, sumatriptan by subcutaneous injection can abort attack in most patients. The obsession and paranoia, as well as hallucinations, should be considered unusual in cluster headaches. Headache specialists I talked to felt that *Pi* is a great movie and a teaching example of cluster headache, with its obsessional restlessness and its excruciating pain, and is one of the top films in portrayal of headache.

Many other movies use headache as an affliction associated with deranged characters and major personality disorders. Another key movie is *White Heat* (1949) ⏴, in which James Cagney plays the not suffer fools gladly Cody. According to film critic David Thomson, this noir film fits well into the postwar zeitgeist when screenwriters were interested in the maddening effects of shell shock and other war atrocities. Cody has two major headache attacks. It is told that he initially made up fake headaches to get his mother's attention, but then the headaches become real. His headache starts abruptly, and he falls to the floor grabbing his head. It lasts for about a minute and then subsides when his mother massages his neck. He needs some time to recover, and his mother says, "Do not let them see you like that." Once in jail, he has a second similar attack and again gets an occipital massage. The headache of Cody here is linked to violent and homicidal behavior, and two psychiatrists tell him to go to a mental institution to take care of his headache. He is put in a straitjacket following a major outburst in jail after he hears that his mother has died. We also learn that his father and brother were in an insane asylum. The headache depiction is reasonably certain to be a cluster headache, quickly subsiding with some postictal deterioration. The link to criminal behavior is notable but wrong.

Another interesting film depicting migraine is *Gods and Monsters* (1998) ⏴⏴, where the protagonist has a severe unilateral headache, nearly collapses, grabs his head, and next is found lying in a chair. His caretaker runs to him with a large assortment of pills, and he asks for luminal. A consulted physician (perhaps a neurologist) calls it "stroke" or "electrical activity," but he does not know how to deal with the "killing" headaches.

The film *That Beautiful Somewhere* (2006) shows one of the leading actress (Jane McGregor) with severe migraine. We see her groping for her head and moving around, crying out in pain and also trying a drill on her temporal lobe (identical to in *Pi*, but with no trephination). She walks around in the movie mostly wearing dark-colored glasses.

Quotable Lines of Dialogue

White Heat

Cody — *[Headache] is like a red-hot buzz saw inside my head.*

That Beautiful Somewhere

Catherine — *Pain makes you do things, makes you submit and pray for anything to stop it.*

A thunderclap headache is depicted in *Hannah Arendt* (2012). Her husband Heinrich Blucher (Axel Milberg) suddenly collapses after a severe orbital headache. It is suggested that he has "a brain aneurysm." She visits him in the hospital and tells him, "I spoke to the doctor. He said you only have a fifty percent chance," to which he answers, "Don't forget the other fifty percent." He is seen in a few scenes later without any deficits, calling it "a slight collapse."

The characteristics of headaches in film have been reviewed by Vargas, and it is found that most actors playing headache sufferers were men with characters between the ages of 18 and 49, nearly half of them died from violent attacks, including suicide. A large number of headaches in the movies do have an underlying cause, with about one-third being the result of a tumor or foreign body or toxic exposure.

A Final Word

Headache is common in the movies, but mostly it is only very briefly mentioned and rarely (except for *Pi*) advances the narrative. It is briefly mentioned with brain tumors or incidentally used, and its function in the plot is often not exactly clear. For screenwriters it may be simply that bad and shady characters should have torturous headaches. Migraine, despite its common occurrence, does not seem to interest screenwriters and its common benign nature is not dramatic enough.

Further Reading

Ashkenazi A, Schwedt T. Cluster headache—Acute and prophylactic therapy. *Headache* 2011;51:272–86.
Nesbitt AD, Goadsby PJ. Cluster headache. *BMJ* 2012;344:e2407.
Pietrobon D, Moskowitz MA. Pathophysiology of migraine. *Annu Rev Physiol* 2013;75:365–91.
Thomson D. *Moments that made the movies*. New York: Thames and Hudson, 2013.
Vargas BB, Henry KA, Boylan LS. Characteristics of headache in motion pictures: Demographics and outcomes of headache sufferers in film. *American Headache Society 49th Annual Scientific Meeting*. Chicago, IL, 2007.

SLEEP DISORDERS IN FILM

Side Effects (2013); starring Rooney Mara, Jude Law, Catherine Zeta-Jones, and Channing Tatum; directed by Steven Soderbergh, written by Scott Z. Burns; distributed by Open Roads Films.

Rating

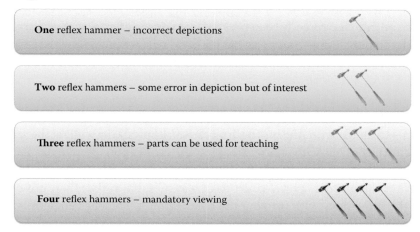

One reflex hammer – incorrect depictions

Two reflex hammers – some error in depiction but of interest

Three reflex hammers – parts can be used for teaching

Four reflex hammers – mandatory viewing

Criticism and Context

Sleep disorders is an interesting chapter in neurologic portrayal in the movies. One should not be surprised to find the common use of dreams and night terrors, and directors have used some specific disorders. Sleepwalking, or somnambulism, is occasionally portrayed in film and often with an erotic undertone. Sleepwalking is most comically displayed in Hal Roach's *High and Dizzy* (1920) ⚒. Harold Lloyd as "the boy" watches Mildred Davis as "the girl" sleepwalking on a building's ledge. (The origin of this absurd sleepwalking posture—outstretched arm(s), eyes closed, and sometimes marching like walking—is not known, but it has made its way into many art forms.) He saves her from falling and places her on a bed. She caresses his face but is startled after she discovers having him in her bedroom.

Bunuel's *Viridiana* (1961) ⚒, banned by the Spanish government due to obscenity and blasphemy, has Viridiana (a nun) dressed in a nightgown sleepwalk, showing off her legs. She is terribly embarrassed that her uncle did not wake her up (he suggests it is dangerous).

Sleepwalking is prominently on display in a newer film, *Side Effects* (2013). *Side Effects* also has an associated website (www.tryablixa.com) that is eerily similar to a real advertisement until Jude Law shows up as the psychiatrist, Dr. Jonathan Banks. He asks questions about signs of depression. If all three questions are answered "yes," he is very concerned and suggests Ablixa. If all three questions are answered "no," he still recommends a referral to a psychiatrist. It seems hard to "escape" a psychiatrist, let alone "Ablixa" (a fictitious antidepressant).

The drug Ablixa, in the main character, causes violent sleepwalking. Emily Taylor (Rooney Mara) is hopelessly depressed, possibly set off by her husband, who has recently been released from prison after serving 4 years for insider trading. Emily tries to get her life back together but fails with the first social encounter. Next she purposely drives her car into the wall of a parking garage, and hospitalization leads to therapy sessions with Dr. Jonathan Banks (Jude Law). He starts prescribing multiple antidepressants, and eventually, when all else fails—and after another attempt to throw herself under a train—treats her with Ablixa. The drug causes sleepwalking while at the same time furnishes her with a cure. Stopping the medication, despite the seemingly innocent act of brief sleepwalking, is not an option she will consider.

After the murder, a brief court drama ensues, but rather than presenting the difficulties with proving the relationship of violent behavior with sleepwalking, this segment ends quickly. It is mentioned that consciousness provides a context for our actions, and that awareness does not exist when you sleep. The film does not mention video-EEG-polysomnographic assessment and its potential value in court. The case quickly goes to a plea bargain, case closed.

Dr. Banks's psychiatry practice suffers; his marriage almost falls apart; and he is grilled in a deposition asking about his workload and whether he can handle it. His colleague psychiatrists threaten to ostracize him for losing patients.

The film has other not-so-subtle themes and shows psychiatrists talking about medication options (the try-this-in-your-patient-because-it-worked-well-in-mine argument) and cavalierly prescribing for family members. (He gives his wife a beta blocker, and she suggests that there are advantages of having a husband who can provide medication.) Even Dr. Banks's decision to come to the United States is used to imply that patients in the United Kingdom who take medication are sick, while those who take medication in the United States are getting better. It further caricaturizes a lavish lifestyle of specialists, among other unsympathetic portrayals.

The film claims that violent behaviors during sleep can be caused by antidepressants, an exceedingly uncommon side effect. Violent behaviors during sleep are well known and may have dramatic implications, including homicide, nonfatal assaults, but also sexual misconduct. Sleepwalking is usually benign in children, but in adults it can become quite harmful, with not only destruction of property, but also serious injury to bed partners or others. Sexsomnia is a form of parasomnia characterized by atypical and often violent or injuring sexual behavior during sleep. The

American Academy of Sleep Medicine has clear criteria for somnambulism that include persistence of sleep or impaired judgment during ambulation and a disturbance that is not better explained by other disorders, drug use, or substance-use disorder. A recent textbook of sleep medicine mentions that sleep specialists are increasingly asked to evaluate potential court cases where violent behavior might be the result of a sleep disorder. Connecting violence with an underlying sleep disorder is far more difficult, though the literature suggest some criteria such as: (1) previous episodes and documented sleep disorder, (2) arousal stimulus, (3) no attempt to escape, (4) horror of and amnesia for the event, and (5) precipitating factors such as recent sleep deprivation and newly introduced medication.

In *Side Effects*, neurologists may see a sense of truthfulness, and the bland emotion of such an act is very well portrayed. This film is a good example of how psychiatry and neurology may intersect and how sleepwalking-associated murder is linked with real astonishment in the perpetrator.

Rooney Mara plays a very convincing sleepwalker. Sleepwalking shows her putting on music and setting a table (a common occurrence in real-life situations) and waking up her husband. She walks and acts like an automaton. Her eyes-open blank look while performing some detailed task is well depicted. In the key scene, she ends up committing a murder (not a spoiler here, as the crime is already implied in the first minute of the film and prominently present in the trailer). This sets off the film's narrative, but *Side Effects* is one of those films in which nobody is what they seem.

Side Effects, therefore, brings to the forefront an interesting and disturbing phenomenon. That in itself makes the film worth watching, but in the end, *Side Effects* is a thriller—with greed and conceit as a leading motif.

Quotable Lines of Dialogue

Side Effects	
Attorney	*What you're saying is that to have intent you must also have consciousness.*
Dr. Banks	*Consciousness provides a context or meaning for our actions. If that part of you does not exist, then basically we are functioning much like an insect where you just respond instinctively without a thought what your actions mean.*
Attorney	*That part "provides meaning to action"...does that exist when we are asleep?*
Dr. Banks	*No.*

Sleepwalking is only one aspect of the depiction of sleep disorders in film. Dreams and nightmares are omnipresent in cinema. Dreams are often effectively used to create a certain mood, to add a surprising twist, or to unveil a suppressed memory. Even wild awakening from a terrifying dream and finding that the reality is similar is used with much effect in *Take Shelter* (2011). The most phantasmagorical depiction of dreams is in *Inception* (2010), showing a dream within a dream—within a dream.

Nightmares have been effectively used in the classics of cinema and include most memorably the dream sequence featuring Dali-designed psychoanalytic symbols in *Spellbound* (1945). Particularly gripping for physicians is the unsettling nightmarish examination of Professor Isak Borg in the Ingmar Bergman-directed *Wild Strawberries* (1957). Herein, in one of his frequent dreams, he has to redo a bacteriology exam but cannot see what is under the microscope and not only fails, but is graded as incompetent—a grade that ends his medicine studies.

Other common sleep disorders depicted in film are narcolepsy and insomnia. Insomnia is characteristically defined as difficulty initiating sleep and inability to have restorative sleep and, as a result, may increase the risk of daytime accidents and a later risk of depressive illness. The twilight state with lack of sleep has been used repeatedly but with little insight on why it can occur and what its consequences are. *Insomnia* (2002) uses lack of sleep and exhaustion as a result of perpetual daylight in Alaska as a plot device.

The Machinist (2004) ⋖ takes the problems with insomnia even further and is more absurd. The main character in this film (played by Christian Bale) is almost moribundly skinny from lack of sleep (a full year!). Lack of sleep is also causing paranoid behavior.

Narcolepsy and narcoleptic hallucinations are well depicted in *My Own Private Idaho* (1991) ⋘. In this movie, River Phoenix plays a gay street hustler with multiple cataleptic attacks. Here the narcoleptic attacks are triggered by anything that reminds him of his mother and his abandonment as a child. Most hallucinations here are vivid prior childhood memories, presented as old Super-8 films. Most narcoleptic hallucinations are simple acoustic (sound or melody) or simple visual (objects or circles). Hallucination of a person may occur, too, and in this film it is often the face of his mother. These hallucinations are then followed by eyelid quivering and prolonged unconsciousness. In reality, cataplectic attacks are brief but may last for 30 minutes; therefore, the prolonged attacks in this film are incorrectly represented. Here, they seem to be a combination of long cataleptic attacks in combination with signs of sleep paralysis. In other situations, narcoleptic patients may notice that while falling asleep or coming out of sleep they are unable to move, speak, or open their eyes; but this lasts no more than a few minutes. The International Classification of Sleep Disorders includes two forms: narcolepsy with cataplexy and narcolepsy without cataplexy. Finally, cataplexy is shown in an exaggerated manner in the film *Deuce Bigelow* (1999), with an actress dropping to the ground like a stone in contrast to the actual typical slow loss of muscle tone.

Quotable Lines of Dialogue

My Own Private Idaho	
Friends	*I am surprised he can even exist like this on narcolepsy.*
	He is not dead. He is just passed out, and it is a condition.

A Final Word

Normally, sleep should provide rest, and when we have a dream it does not make much sense but, alas, not in the movies. For screenwriters, there is a good reason to use dream sequences and sleep disorders because they love the ethereal dream, particularly night terrors, and because they are a good storytelling device. Sleepwalking is now correctly on display—although in its most severe and rare form.

Further Reading

Kryger MH, Roth T, Dement WC. *Principles and Practice of Sleep Medicine.* Philadelphia: Saunders, 2010.

Siclari F, Khatami R, Urbaniok F, et al. Violence in sleep. *Brain* 2010;133:3494–3509.

Sutcliffe JG, de Lecea L. Not asleep, not quite awake. *Nat Med* 2004;10:673–74.

Zadra A, Desautels A, Petit D, Montplaisir J. Somnambulism: Clinical aspects and pathophysiological hypotheses. *Lancet Neurol* 2013;12:285–94.

SEIZURES IN FILM

A Matter of Life and Death (1946); David Niven, Roger Livesey, Raymond Massey, Kim Hunter, and Marius Goring; written and directed by Michael Powell and Emeric Pressburger; distributed by Eagle Lion Films.

Rating

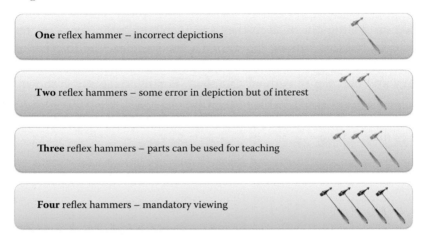

One reflex hammer – incorrect depictions

Two reflex hammers – some error in depiction but of interest

Three reflex hammers – parts can be used for teaching

Four reflex hammers – mandatory viewing

Criticism and Context

One of the best-analyzed films on seizures is *A Matter of Life and Death*, also known as *Stairway to Heaven*. The story line is complex and fantastical. It involves an RAF pilot (David Niven) who survives a plane crash. He has fallen in love with an American radio operator whom he talked to just before the crash, and has reunited with her and is deeply in love. Under normal circumstances, he would have died and would have appeared in heaven, but the film shows him not checking in. The story then turns to a heavenly tribunal discussing his failure to arrive in heaven and whether falling in love on earth is sufficient to postpone death.

Several chapters during the film show he has spells that may be interpreted as complex partial seizures. The spells are stereotyped and always begin with a smell of fried onions or with a discordant piano piece followed by visions of a "heavenly conductor" and more complex hallucinations of a stairway to heaven to the aforementioned tribunal, where he eventually may have to defend his stay on Earth.

A neurosurgeon appears and Dr. Reeves is able to examine him during a spell, and a pupil abnormality and possible Babinski sign is found. Dr. Reeves's diagnosis is "fine vascular meningeal adhesions binding the optic nerve to the brain, the internal carotid artery, similar adhesions in chiasm and the brain." He is rushed into surgery and even has a spell under full anesthesia, where the key scene eventually depicts the tribunal arguing his stay on Earth or need to come to heaven. (He wins his case and stays.)

Quotable Lines of Dialogue

A Matter of Life and Death	
Dr. Reeves	*He is having a series of highly organized hallucinations comparable to an experience of actual life, a combination of vision, hearing, and of ideas. To a neurologist, that compares to a direct sense of smell and taste. Once that connection is established, we know to look for the trouble.*

A Matter of Life and Death has been analyzed in detail by psychologist David Friedman (1992), who makes a persuasive case of complex partial seizures. The film is obviously exaggerated. One of the film's strengths is the depiction of a complex seizure. However, visual hallucinations are never that complex or as detailed, and they never present as a full nightmare; but some of it indeed may indicate a temporal lobe lesion. (None of that is clear, and Dr. Reeves's localization is way off.) No other film has depicted temporal lobe epilepsy well (see Chapter 6 for violence and temporal lobe epilepsy).

Epilepsy in film has been well studied, and different types have even been acted out (Table 3.2). Much credit should be given to psychologist Sallie Baxendale (2003), who analyzed 62 films, concluding that there were "examples of all of the ancient beliefs surrounding epilepsy such as demonic or divine possession, genius, lunacy, delinquency, and general otherness." A link between epilepsy and psychiatry often implied that male characters were mad, bad, and dangerous. Female characters with seizures were exotic and vulnerable. In some films, the protagonist has seizures, but rarely does a seizure disorder drive the full narrative. A recent film from India, *Ek Naya Din* (*A New Day*) (2013), got attention when it emphasized bad spirits in epilepsy and treatment with witchcraft. The neurologist,

TABLE 3.2   Types of Epilepsy Depicted in Film

Epilepsy and violence	*Deceiver* (1997)
Posttraumatic epilepsy	*The Winning Team* (1952)
Photosensitive epilepsy	*The Andromeda Strain* (1971)
Epilepsy surgery (hemispherectomy)	*The Other Half of Me* (2001)
Epilepsy (ketogenic diet)	*First Do No Harm* (1997)
Pseudoseizures	*Drugstore Cowboy* (1989)
Stress convulsions	*Black Hawk Down* (2001)
Side effects of antipsychotic drugs	*Take Shelter* (2012)

Misra, created this movie to improve understanding. Illiteracy and superstition are prevalent in north India, where tremendous poverty coexists.

Several other films are noteworthy. In *Frankie and Johnny* (1991) ⋞, a man has a seizure in a restaurant—"a fit or something"—and Frankie (Michelle Pfeiffer) puts him on his side while in a postictal period. She sees that he has a necklace that says epilepsy. While they are waiting for the ambulance, Johnny (Al Pacino) asks her out, but she is not interested. The man awakens rapidly and asks what happened, and Johnny answers, "Nothing much. I just got turned down by someone."

Pseudoseizures are most prominent in *Drugstore Cowboy* (1989) ⋘. Here pseudoseizures are deliberate, and in the film the "seizing" person takes Alka-Seltzer to fake foaming at the mouth (a clever find from the director). The attention to the "seizing" person allows others to steal prescription drugs in the drugstore. The psychogenic seizure is surprisingly accurately done, with thrashing movements, moaning, and eyes closed shut. When it is over, she suddenly walks away with bystanders asking, "Are you okay?" A pseudoseizure is also seen in *The Intouchables* (2012), where it also has a deliberate deceiving purpose.

Although initially made for TV (and therefore outside the scope of this book), *First Do No Harm* (1997) ⋞ is a movie made by Jim Abrahams who had a "similar" experience with his son, Charlie. (He is the founder of the Charlie Foundation.) The film is interesting because of its comprehensive coverage of childhood epilepsy. Meryl Streep plays a desperate mother whose son (Fred Ward) has epilepsy. The movie does not hold back and has caricatured all that may go wrong with epilepsy—arrogant neurologists failing to accept ketogenic diet as a viable alternative, Stevens-Johnson syndrome from antiepileptic drugs, paraldehyde brought in a styrofoam cup showing the cup melting away from direct drug exposure, behavior problems with antiepileptic drugs, and even seizure on an airplane. To top it off, the movie even has a discussion on lack of randomized trials in epilepsy treatment and thus sufficient reason to try more experimental approaches—the "if you think this approach does not work, where is the proof of your approach" argument. All is well with the child after a ketogenic diet is started.

Even the separate stages of seizures are shown in film, but rarely accurately. Postictal confusion is never depicted in Robert Altman's *A Wedding* (1978). There is immediate recovery after what seems a generalized tonic clonic seizure. The aura in *The Aura* (2005) ⋘ is about the protagonist, who has epilepsy. The aura is described in a lengthy scene and is used to profoundly scare the listener. It goes as follows: "There is a moment, a shift…things suddenly change; it is as if everything stops, a door opens in your head that lets things in—sounds, voices, images, smells. Smells from school, kitchen, and family. Cannot move. It is horrible and perfect." The aura is further accompanied by a screeching horror sound followed by a black screen and awakening with bright light shining in his eyes. The aura here creates a sense of mysticism. It conforms to the general impression that screenwriters think that seizures are a harbinger of doom.

A Final Word

Seizures are common in the movies, and understandably so. Similarly, as in the real world, their presentation might be frightening and this opportunity for drama has been noted by screenwriters. A wide variety of causes for seizures has been depicted, but many of them occur in stressful situations. It is very obvious that seizures in film are linked to madness, perpetuating the age-old myth of a link between seizures and psychiatric disorders. Readers interested in the historical significance of seizures may seek out *Cleopatra* (1963), where Caesar (Richard Burton) proclaims, "One day it will happen where I cannot hide, where the world shall see me fail…. I shall foam at the mouth and they will tear me to pieces."

Further Reading

Baxendale S. Epilepsy at the movies: Possession to presidential assassination. *Lancet Neurol* 2003;2:764–70.

Christie I. *A matter of life and death.* London: British Film Institute, 2000.

Friedman DB. A matter of fried onions. *Seizure* 1992;1:307–10.

Kerson JF, Kerson TS, Kerson LA. The depiction of seizures in film. *Epilepsia* 1999;40:1163–67.

Sharma DC. Indian film on epilepsy busts myths. *Lancet Neurol* 2013;3:245.

CEREBRAL PALSY IN FILM

Gaby: A True Story (1987); starring Rachel Levin, Norma Aleandro, Liv Ullmann, and Robert Loggia; directed by Luis Madoki, written by Martin Salinas and Michael James Love; Academy Award and a Golden Globe for best supporting actress (Norma Aleandro); distributed by TriStar Pictures.

Rating

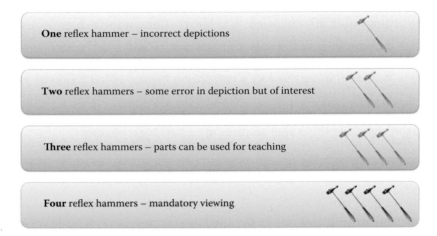

My Left Foot (1989); starring Daniel Day-Lewis, Ray McAnally, Brenda Fricker, Fiona Shaw, and Hugh O'Conor; written and directed by Jim Sheridan; Academy Award for best actor (Daniel Day-Lewis) and best actress in a supporting role (Brenda Fricker); distributed by Granada Films and Miramax.

Rating

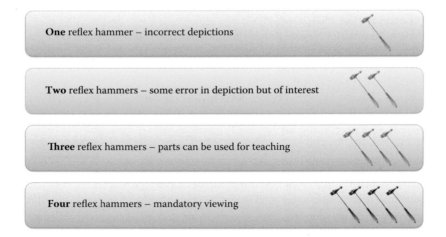

Criticism and Context

Cerebral palsy is a brain injury that is mostly established before birth and can dramatically impact a person's functioning and activities. One of the first major feature films to address this issue was *Gaby: A True Story*, which described the upbringing and development of the Mexican writer Gabriela Brimmer. The original book is authored in three voices told by Gaby, her mother, Sari, and her caregiver, Florencia Morales Sánchez. Gaby became the leading figure of Mexican people with disabilities; she died at the age of 52 in 2000.

Quotable Lines of Dialogue

Gaby: A True Story	
Gaby	*How can I scream when I can't talk?*
	God, if life is so many things that I am not, and never will be, give me the strength to be what I am.
	How can I stop loving with the seed of a woman inside me?

Norma Aleandro, who plays Gaby, mostly acts out manifestations of chorea but shows no signs of pseudobulbar palsy. In the beginning of the film, the family is incorrectly told that cerebral palsy is a consequence of Rhesus incompatibility and that she can be mentally retarded or "locked inside her body." Her mother, played by Liv Ullmann, plays a somewhat remote role, but not her nanny, Florencia, who acts as an interpreter. The nanny is the one who first discovers that Gaby can communicate using her feet. At 8 years old, she enters a rehabilitation center's elementary school. There her language arts teacher persuades her to write. As readers of this book have noticed by now, it is not surprising that this film also includes sexual awakening, once she falls in love with a disabled schoolmate. There is some insight into the disability with cerebral palsy, but the film is easily overshadowed by *My Left Foot*.

The film *My Left Foot* is painstakingly crafted and represents cerebral palsy played by Hugh O'Conor as young Christy Brown and Daniel Day-Lewis as adult Christy Brown. The film opens with him at a charity and then flashes back to his birth. ("Your son has been born. There have been some complications.") The film (inaccurately) suggests a fetal anoxic event during labor, but the onset of this static lesion of the cerebral motor cortex is unknown. Very few cases of cerebral palsy are likely to have severe acute hypoxia during birth. Multiple births, maternal infection antepartum, vaginal bleeding, and fetal infection are all risk factors, but the prevalence is very low. The diagnosis of cerebral palsy is based on a major manifestation of spasticity coexisting with dystonia. The film suggests that psychotherapy and occupational and speech therapy could be applied successfully, but there is little evidence these help. In some children, motor skills improve. Long-term effects are common, including joint dislocation, scoliosis, and deformities.

Christy Brown came from a family of 13 children, and his mother taught him to write and paint. Dublin in the 1930s housed working people and the poor in large sections of town. Children with disabilities would go to "a home," and there were no facilities. The Catholic Church provided shelter and food to the poor but had no practical solution to severe disability. Christy was born under problematic circumstances and apparently was unresponsive after birth and floppy. His mother knew he was different, but she also knew that there was more inside and therefore taught him. According to his biographer, Anthony Jordan, "Every spare moment she had was spent trying to communicate with her son, trying to unlock the brain she knew was within the twisted frame." The film shows the first discovery of intelligence when he is able to write he could write the letter "A" on a chalkboard. The film clearly shows many community members having a fixed presumption about major cognitive deficits, labeling them as instances of major mental retardation.

Quotable Lines of Dialogue

My Left Foot	
Man in bar	*Are you gonna put him in a home, Paddy?*
Paddy Brown	*I'll go in a coffin before any son of mine will go in a home.*
Man in bar	*Now, Paddy, I believe it's the end of the road.*
Woman	*And there he was lyin' at the bottom of the stairs like a moron.*
Priest	*You can get out of purgatory, but you can never get out of hell. He's a terrible cross to the poor woman.*

Daniel Day-Lewis (Figure 3.9) is incomparable in depicting cerebral palsy with its pseudobulbar signs and dystonic postures and avoids the so-common overplaying of grimacing. The uncontrollable outbursts of screaming and crying may seem a bit unrealistic, but some outbursts like this may occur in real life under circumstances of stress. The happy ending of marrying his nurse in the film should be contrasted to the real Christy Brown (Figure 3.9), who became an alcoholic (some of it is shown in the film having him drink from a straw out of a bottle hidden in his pocket).

Christy Brown's book *My Left Foot* was followed by *Down All the Days*, an autobiographical work about living in the slums of Dublin in the first part of the twentieth century. The book showed drink and violence, but also hopelessness and recklessness. ("We are all jarred, Christy, you know. You're not the only one. We all need a bit of help.") It has been speculated that his tremendous unchanneled urge and energy and frustration may have resulted in depression and alcoholism. He married Mary Carr, who neglected him. He apparently died when he choked on a lamb chop.

The movie shows Christy's relationship with Dr. Collis, who became the founder of Cerebral Palsy Ireland. Dr. Collis developed a specific program in training and movement and generally getting the athetoid to work in whatever position was easiest. This was usually the sleeping posture. Speech therapy would provide control of the respiratory muscle and swallowing muscle.

Christy also joined the New Association for Disabled Artists and began painting. He did painting tours and exhibitions throughout Ireland. A major problem was Christy's alcohol abuse, and this also affected his writing and output. According to his biographer, A.J. Jordan, he was "erudite and a philosophical man, who endured a long apprenticeship; but when success did come, he succeeded to 'Vanity Fair.'"

Two other films on cerebral palsy should be mentioned. *Oasis* (2002) portrays an abandoned young woman with cerebral palsy and a complicated courtship. The correct display of dystonia and spastic dysphonia won Moon So-Ri a Best Actress award at the Venice Film Festival. She is constantly grunting, in spasm, with eyes turning, and grimacing. The film is also unique because there are several scenes where she has fantasies of being normal and not spastic. This may occur in patients with cerebral palsy, but the desire to be considered normal is more often seen in patients with much less severe manifestations. *Door to Door* (2002) was a TV film in the United States that gained prominence because of its theme of

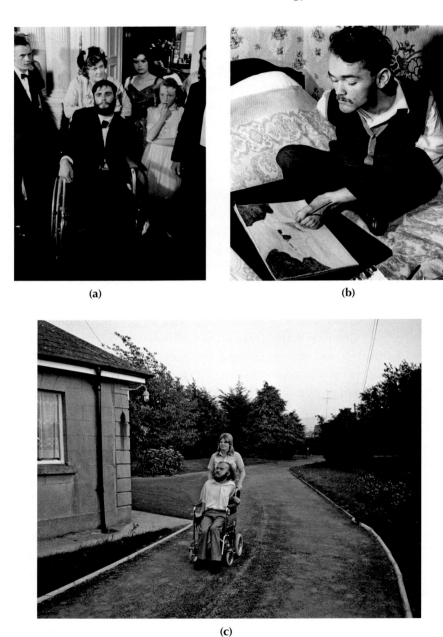

FIGURE 3.9 (a) Daniel Day-Lewis playing Christy Brown; (b) Christy Brown painting with his left foot; (c) Christy Brown in later life. (Used with permission of Irish Photo Archives and Ferndale Films/Hells Kitchen and Getty Images.)

persistence. It is based on the true story of Bill Porter, a door-to-door salesman who could not drive well, speak well, and walked clumsily as a result of a "mild" cerebral palsy. These skills are needed for any door-to-door salesman, but he muscled through. (In real life, he was the top salesman for the grocery he worked for.) The film stars William H. Macy, who accurately plays his challenge—walking up to 10 miles daily and selling almost anything to everybody. This comparatively mild case of cerebral palsy is poorly acted with unusual distorted faces, unlike Daniel Day-Lewis, and is of little interest.

A Final Word

Several films portray the major physical disability of cerebral palsy. The films celebrate creativity and normal intelligence. Many of those affected by cerebral palsy are wrongly considered mentally handicapped. It is good to see that this topic has interested directors.

Further Reading

Agarwal A, Verma I. Cerebral palsy in children: An overview. *J Clinical Orthopaedics Trauma* 2012;3:77–81.

Aisen ML, Kerkovich D, Mast J, et al. Cerebral palsy: Clinical care and neurological rehabilitation. *Lancet Neurol* 2011;10:844–52.

Bax MC, Flodmark O, Tydeman C. Definition and classification of cerebral palsy: From syndrome toward disease. *Dev Med Child Neurol Suppl* 2007;109:39–41.

Collis WR, O'Donnell M. Cerebral palsy. *Arch Dis Child* 1951;26:387–98.

Hambleton GL. *Christy Brown: The life that inspired* My Left Foot. Edinburgh: Mainstream Publishing, 2012.

Jordan AJ. *Christy Brown's omen: A biography drawing on his letters*, incorporating *Founding of cerebral palsy Ireland* by R. Collis. Dublin: Westport Books, 1998.

McIntyre S, Taitz D, Keogh J, et al. A systematic review of risk factors for cerebral palsy in children born at term in developed countries. *Dev Med Child Neurol* 2013;55:499–508.

AUTISM SPECTRUM DISORDERS IN FILM

Fly Away (2011); starring Beth Broderick, Ashley Rickards, and Greg Germann; written and directed by Janet Grillo; distributed by New Video Group.

Rating

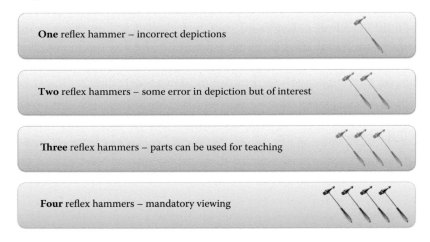

Adam (2009); starring Hugh Dancy, Rose Byrne, and Frankie Faison; written and directed by Max Mayer; won Alfred P. Sloan Prize at Sundance Film Festival; distributed by Fox Searchlight Pictures.

Rating

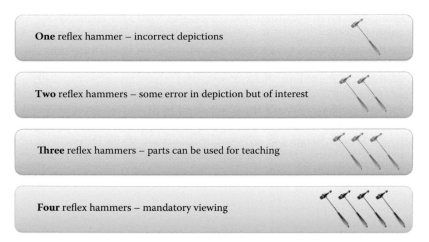

Criticism and Context

Autism spectrum disorders are present in nearly 1 in 70 US children. There are many specialized autism clinics in the United States, and these disorders require a multidisciplinary evaluation and mostly include neurologists. For many viewers, *Rain Man* (1988) ⁓ is the key movie portraying autism, but not to experts in the field. Most criticize the film for suggesting that autism is associated with savant syndrome (hyper-systemizing, presence of a memory brilliance), which it is not, or rarely so. Dustin Hoffman's mannerisms feel contrived, and it is sentimentality that wins. Pauline Kael—one of the most revered film critics—called it "wet kitsch."

After *Rain Man*, films appeared with a more differentiated depiction of autism. *Fly Away* is largely about the acceptance of Jeanne (Beth Broderick) that her autistic teenage daughter Mandy needs help and cannot stay in her current social environment. Her attacks are muted by the lullaby "Lady Bug, Lady Bug, Fly Away." The film shows an extreme behavior disorder attributed to autism, with Mandy screaming and attacking other children at school and at playgrounds. The mother, Jeanne, is completely overwhelmed, burned out, and beaten up, living in a messy house. Mandy is a frightening child, and Jeanne is the persevering mother who endures against all odds.

Quotable Lines of Dialogue

Fly Away	
Schoolteacher	*Realistically we have to provide her with skills.*
Mother	*Skills?… Like pushing a broom?*
Schoolteacher	*If it makes her feel good?*
Mother	*Mandy is smart. Inside all of that, she is so smart. Just because you cannot handle it, it does not mean my daughter belongs in an institution.*
Schoolteacher	*If you want to play the martyr, that is your choice, not mine.*

The movie has little to say about autism, but Mandy's moments of quiet drawing followed by night terrors are real. There is a continuous refusal by Jeanne to find a better solution. Because Mandy's flailing around in a car nearly causes an accident, it leads to her being transferred to a residential home for autistic children.

Autism spectrum disorders include Asperger's syndrome, and the differences between these disorders are shown in Table 3.3. The films *Adam* and *Extremely Loud & Incredibly Close* (2011) deal with Asperger's syndrome. Both display repetitive behaviors and fixation on topics.

TABLE 3.3   Differential Diagnostic Features of Autism Spectrum Disorders

Features	Autism	Asperger's syndrome
Age of recognition (diagnosis) [a]	0–3 years (3–5 years)	>3 years (6–8 years)
Regression	About 25% (social or communication)	No
Sex ratio (male:female)	2:1	4:1
Socialization	Poor	Poor
Communication	Delayed, might be nonverbal	No early delay; qualitative and pragmatic difficulties later
Behavior	More impaired than in Asperger's syndrome	Variable (circumscribed interests)
Intellectual disability	>60%	Mild to none
Cause	More likely to establish genetic or other cause than in Asperger's syndrome	Variable
Seizures	Experienced by 25% over life span	Experienced by roughly 10% over life span
Outcome	Poor to fair	Fair to good

[a] Data adapted from Volkmar, FR and Pauls D. Autism. *Lancet* 2003;362:1133–41.

Adam very specifically addresses the social interactions and relationship problems people have with these autism spectrum disorders or, as the character of Beth says in the movie, "not prime relationship material." Adam is preoccupied with the solar system and the universe, and conversations often start with minute numerical details of the Big Bang and later expansion of the universe. He tells his girlfriend Beth (Rose Byrne) that his brain works differently than "neurotypicals." Examples of problematic behavior are many and include applying for nearly 100 jobs after getting laid off and being unable to go to a restaurant and eat something different than macaroni and cheese on a daily basis. Adam is angry with Beth's father, leading to a major confrontation and the couple finally breaking up. Beth gives him chocolates after this because she feels sorry, and he responds, "I am not Forrest Gump." The disorder is accurately presented as a social interaction problem with outbursts of anger when his world is rocked. He is not able to handle such situations well.

Quotable Lines of Dialogue

Adam

| Adam | *Their sensor systems have detected an error in analyzing space.* |
| Friend | *Adam, I am having lunch. Speak English. No more black holes, black hole radiation, Mars robots. Lunch time is for guys talking about women, the weather, and such.* |

The thin line between a nerd and being afflicted by Asperger's syndrome is clear in *Napoleon Dynamite* (2004). In a film showing features of teen culture and bullying, Napoleon is a social misfit. Psychiatrists Levin and Schlozman (2006) have argued he has a socially disconnected character but may have symptoms consistent with Asperger's syndrome. There is impairment of nonverbal behavior (facing the floor when speaking), abruptly stopping conversations, irritability, and dysphonia. However, some people have strongly argued that Napoleon could belong to "geekdom" and nothing more.

Autism has become more prevalent over the last 10 years (partly as a result of better recognition). It is rarely (<10%) associated with a severe disorder such as tuberous sclerosis, fragile X, or fetal alcohol syndrome. The association of autism and MMR vaccine has been consistently denied by most experts. Volumetric studies and neurotransmitters have been studied, and some abnormalities have been found, but most MRIs in children diagnosed with autism are normal.

A Final Word

Autism spectrum disorders have long been considered disorders that may rarely cross the specialty of neurology, but recent work has identified that an anatomical substrate is likely. The above-mentioned films have used this disability to fill an entire screenplay, and the portrayal is generally accurate and can be used for teaching.

Further Reading

Levin HW, Schlozman S. *Napoleon Dynamite*: Asperger's disorder or Geek NOS? *Acad Psychiatry* 2006;30:430–35.

Levy SE, Mandell DS, Schultz RT. Autism. *Lancet* 2009;374:1627–38.

Manning-Courtney P, Murray D, Currans K, et al. Autism spectrum disorders. *Curr Probl Pediatr Adolesc Health Care* 2013;43:2–11.

Pellegrino L, Liptak GS. Consultation with the specialist: Asperger syndrome. *Pediatr Rev* 2011;32:481–88; quiz 489.

Volkmar FR, Pauls D. Autism. *Lancet* 2003;362:1133–41.

Yates K, Le Couteur A. Diagnosing autism. *Paediatrics and Child Health* 2013;23:5–10.

Zwaigenbaum L, Bryson S, Garon N. Early identification of autism spectrum disorders. *Behav Brain Res* 2013;251:133–46.

TOURETTE SYNDROME IN FILM

Niagara, Niagara (1997); starring Henry Thomas, Robin Tunney, Michael Parks, and Stephen Lang; directed by Bob Gosse, written by Matthew Weiss; best actress award for Robin Tunney at Venice Film Festival; distributed by Lions Gate Films.

Rating

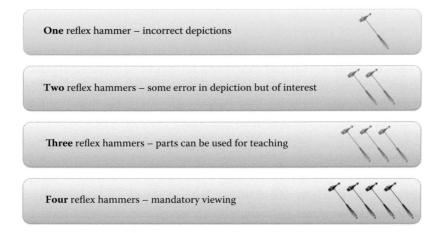

One reflex hammer – incorrect depictions

Two reflex hammers – some error in depiction but of interest

Three reflex hammers – parts can be used for teaching

Four reflex hammers – mandatory viewing

The Tic Code (1997); starring Christopher Marquette, Gregory Hines, and Polly Draper; directed by Gary Winick, written by Polly Draper; Crystal Bear Award at Berlin International Film Festival.

Rating

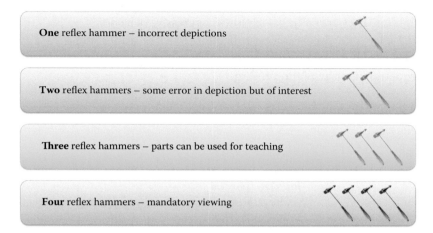

One reflex hammer – incorrect depictions

Two reflex hammers – some error in depiction but of interest

Three reflex hammers – parts can be used for teaching

Four reflex hammers – mandatory viewing

Criticism and Context

Tourette's syndrome is autosomal dominant by complex segregation techniques, but no genome linkage has been found. Treatment is a combination of psychological techniques and pharmacologic management, mostly dopamine antagonists or atypical neuroleptics. Not long ago, Tourette's was seen as a psychiatric disorder and treated with psychotherapy. It is now a reasonably well-treatable medical disorder.

Niagara, Niagara is a love story with an unclear plotline between two misfits. Tourette's plays predominantly in this film and is the basis of violent eruptions, and eventually a fatal outcome. Marcy (Robin Tunney) and Seth (Henry Thomas) meet when they are shoplifting, and their relationship evolves into holdups in drugstores. The film implies that Tourette's syndrome can lead to violent behavior.

Tourette's is shown with phonic tics, and the representation is remarkable. The fact that they occur during times of personal stress is accurate. The common symptoms of echolalia (imitation of sounds of others) or coprolalia (involuntary obscene gestures) are all demonstrated. Marcy explains that all the girls in her grammar school called her nicknames: "Mental Marcy," "Spazzy," "Twitchy." She explains that drinking helps her and "for some reason sex helps." She even discusses incorporating tics into a voluntary movement. At one point, she goes to a drugstore and asks for Haldol and Cogentin (appropriate medication for Tourette's). Symptoms of obsessive-compulsive behavior are shown and explained (repeatedly tapping on her boyfriend and organizing pencils and nail-polish bottles). A major fight breaks out at the end of the film, likely in an effort to show the social difficulties resulting in fistfights. ("They are calling it explosive-aggressive behavior.")

The Tic Code shows uncontrollable facial tics under stress in a film that has a major melodramatic tone. The protagonist, Miles (Christopher Marquette), is a jazz piano prodigy.

Quotable Lines of Dialogue

The Tic Code	
Laura	*I think it means a lot to him to see someone with a similar neurologic problem.*
Tyrone	*Neurologic problem? I heard it called many things but never a neurologic problem.*
Laura	*What do you call it?*
Tyrone	*I call it something I don't like to talk about.*

The movie shows his father's denial in accepting this syndrome as a neurologic disorder. The film becomes a buddy movie when Miles finds a saxophonist with Tourette's syndrome. (The film's screenwriter, Polly Draper, has him modeled after her husband, who has Tourette's.) *The Tic Code* is quite impressive in its portrayal of involuntary (and mostly muted) mimicry. Miles (Chris Marquette) makes guttural repetitive sounds/vocalizations and tries to hold his breath. "I am not holding my breath, just holding my feelings." He is also seen with compulsory touching of objects. He is unable to play when stressed. His father left the family because of his tics, and his mother, Laura (Polly Draper), explains Tourette's as, "He's got a few less inhibitors in his brain."

His father wants a genetic test because his new girlfriend is "creeped out by that Tourette's thing," but he is told angrily by Laura that genetic testing does not exist. Miles is nervous about seeing his father again after many years and puts on a patch (what kind not mentioned, but likely a clonidine patch).

Several other films briefly use Tourette's syndrome. An absurdly funny portrayal is in *Deuce Bigalow: Male Gigolo* (1999) ⌣, where one of the protagonist's female clients has long-lasting major tics and persistent echolalia and coprolalia to humorous effect. Her normal speech is constantly interrupted by sexual verbiage, but Deuce tells her he has a solution. He takes her to a baseball game where the people in the stadium interpret her outbursts as a critique of the game, and the crowd begins to shout out using her same language.

Tics and "hemifacial spasms" are common in Nicolas Cage in *Matchstick Men* (2003) ✕ and are associated with a considerable obsessive-compulsive disorder with compulsions and ritualistic behavior (closing the door three times). Inappropriate vocalizations are also apparent, suggesting Tourette's syndrome; but the full "syndrome" depicted in this film is not easily classifiable.

A Final Word

Gilles de la Tourette's syndrome is rare (worldwide prevalence of 1%), and one would expect that the strange vocalizations such as sniffing, throat clearing, snorting, and tics with twitching and head nodding would be of interest to filmmakers writing comedies. Hollywood's use of this disorder allows the screenwriter to have the character curse and fight whenever it comes in handy. Whether antisocial behavior is related to Tourette's syndrome is a topic of discussion among experts. Severe Tourette's syndrome is rare, and antisocial behavior is uncommon. Perhaps at some point there will be some appreciation of the seriousness of the disorder, its complex presentation, and associated compulsive behavior.

Further Reading

Cavanna AE, Seri S. Tourette's syndrome. *BMJ* 2013;347:f4964.

Knight T, Steeves T, Day L, et al. Prevalence of tic disorders: A systematic review and meta-analysis. *Pediatr Neurol* 2012;47:77–90.

Plessen KJ. Tic disorders and Tourette's syndrome. *Eur Child Adolesc Psychiatry* 2013;22 Suppl 1:S55–60.

Robertson MM. Tourette syndrome, associated conditions and the complexities of treatment. *Brain* 2000;123 Pt 3:425–62.

Robertson MM. The Gilles de la Tourette syndrome: The current status. *Arch Dis Child Educ Pract Ed* 2012;97:166–75.

DEMENTIA IN FILM

Iris (2001); starring Dame Judi Dench, Kate Winslet, Jim Broadbent, and Hugh Bonneville; directed by Richard Eyre, written by Richard Eyre and Charles Wood; BAFTA Award for best actress (Judi Dench), Academy Award and Golden Globe Award for best supporting actor (Jim Broadbent); distributed by Miramax Films.

Rating

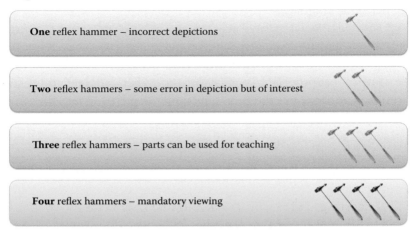

A Song for Martin (En Sång För Martin) (2001); starring Sven Wollter, Viveka Seldahl, and Reine Brynolfsson; directed by Bille August, written by Bille August and Ulla Isaksson; distributed by Film i Väst.

Rating

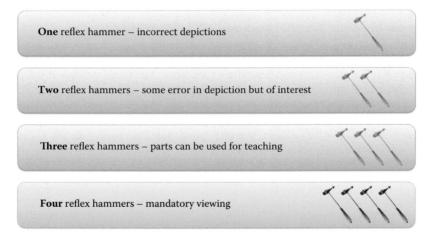

Away from Her (2006); starring Julie Christie, Gordon Pinsent, Olympia Dukakis, and Michael Murphy; directed by Sarah Polley, written by Alice Munro and Sarah Polley; Golden Globe Award and Screen Actors Guild Award for Julie Christie; distributed by Lions Gate Films.

Rating

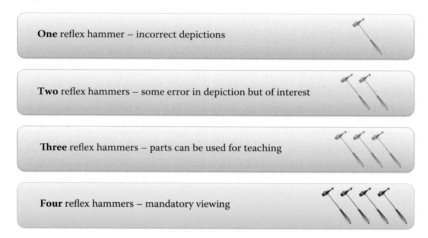

One reflex hammer – incorrect depictions

Two reflex hammers – some error in depiction but of interest

Three reflex hammers – parts can be used for teaching

Four reflex hammers – mandatory viewing

Criticism and Context

Many films unfortunately and inaccurately present a dementing illness as a consequence of old age (*On Golden Pond* [1981], *Agnes of God* [1985]). Some famous actors now are playing themselves as frail octogenarians. (See Jeanne Moreau in *Gebo and the Shadow* [2012] and Jean-Louis Trintignant in *Amour* [2012].) However, there are some remarkable films portraying dementia in the elderly (and also with young age onset).

Iris accurately tells the story of one of the most gifted novelists of the twentieth century, Dame Iris Murdoch. Previously a tutor at St. Anne's College at Oxford, she became a full-time writer producing more than two dozen novels. Her dementia became apparent in 1995 after her last book, *Jackson's Dilemma*. She attributed major problems writing this novel to "writer's block," but in retrospect, there were early red flags. That is the underpinning of this film.

Iris, the film, is about her courtship with John Bayley (played here both by Jim Broadbent and Hugh Bonneville), who would himself write several memoirs. The movie shows the early beginnings of other manifestations of dementia that, in retrospect, were early signs. During a TV interview, she loses her train of thought, is lost for words, and comes home confused and agitated, not remembering details about the interview. The film introduces circumlocutory errors ("It is the man who brings the mail") and inability to name the prime minister. In her cluttered office, she seems to agonize over words ("puzzle is a funny word," to which John answers, "All words are like that when you take them by surprise, aren't they?"). When the general physician arrives, she tells him that writing her new book is very tiring and difficult.

Quotable Lines of Dialogue

Iris	
Neurologist	*What is the name of the prime minister?*
Iris	*Are you asking me? I do not know. Surely it does not matter. Ask John. Someone will know.*

Wandering within and outside the house is shown, and this is a common theme in all films involving dementia. A significant deterioration in sanitation is shown, culminating in placement within a nursing home. John continues to remind her she wrote "novels—wonderful novels." A scene showing her sitting on the beach trying to write notes is allegoric for two reasons. Her diary entries after 1993 were indicative of marked decline, and she won the Man Booker International Prize for her novel *The Sea, The Sea*.

In *A Song for Martin*, the orchestral director and composer first forgets the name of his manager, then confuses the name of his wife with his ex-wife, and, in a poignant scene, has a major derealization episode in the bedroom. He asks his wife to look up signs of cerebral hemorrhage; but because he has no paralysis they conclude it must be something else. He has marked difficulties remembering that night and in his confusion tries hard to get all the details right. The general physician concludes it is overexertion and tells him to slow down. The relentless deterioration is shown with him suddenly forgetting the score while directing the orchestra, and he is embarrassingly led away. He is shown with aggressive outbursts and accusatory behavior, and urinating in a plant container in a restaurant. His wife lovingly copes with his decline but never leaves him alone until institutionalization. The film is a carefully scripted accurate depiction of all phases of Alzheimer's disease. The protagonist shows the dazed and confused behavior and finally emptying of the mind.

A Song for Martin also discusses early management, and the neurologist argues against memantine (NMDA antagonist) and cholinesterase inhibitors (donepezil or rivastigmine) in the early phase, but this would be far easier prescribed in the United States. The neurologist also wrongly mentions reduced cerebral blood flow in explaining Alzheimer's disease, which is an antiquated theory ("cerebrovascular insufficiency"). In clinical practice unfortunately there are still some patients who are prescribed vasodilators with no measurable effect.

The film arguably presents the phases of Alzheimer's disease in a somewhat reversed format. The neurologist diagnoses "incipient Alzheimer's" (now called mild cognitive impairment) when Martin suddenly loses track of an entire musical score. The inability to continue while the orchestra is playing is likely seen more often in advanced Alzheimer's disease, but is used here—I am sure—to obtain major dramatic effect.

Sudden episodes of complete derealization while looking in the mirror are another highly unusual presentation. Alzheimer's disease is slowly progressive, but an early sign is name forgetting. The film is correct in associating name forgetting with work situations and not the more benign name forgetting in social situations. Misplacing objects and inability to find one's way back home are also early signs of Alzheimer's disease. Nonetheless, early-onset Alzheimer's disease may present with behavior or executive dysfunction in one-third of the patients.

Away from Her is of interest because it focuses more on the social conundrum facing spouses. The film shows the indistinguishable progression of Alzheimer's disease, but it is of interest due to the husband's reaction to and final acceptance of his wife's dementia. The film starts with Grant explaining, "I never wanted to be away from her. She had the spark of life." Fiona (Julie Christie) finds out that her memory is failing when she is cross-country skiing and cannot remember where she is. Her husband, Grant (Gordon Pinsent), notices that she puts a frying pan in the freezer. Fiona shows a failing memory and the embarrassment and denial that often accompany these episodes in a very accurate way. Fiona does not know when they bought the cottage, has difficulty finding her coat, and seems to be very aware of her evolving deficit. In fact, she reads a book on Alzheimer's disease, and specifically a chapter on caregivers' burden and how they may have to cope with accusatory behavior ("sounds like a regular marriage").

We are told Fiona is young, and she may be in her mid-60s after marrying early and 45 years of marriage. When she starts wandering, her husband drives through the neighborhood to eventually find her shivering on a bridge. They both seem to realize the time has come for her to go to assisted living. Here she meets another man, and she becomes his caregiver. (The nursing-home staff is not surprised; this happens often.)

The husband visits her often, but her answers are platitudes, and she is not aware of his presence.

Quotable Lines of Dialogue

Away from Her	
Fiona	*Once the idea is gone, everything is gone. I just wander around trying to figure out what it is that was so important earlier.*
Husband	*She is in her own world. Perhaps that is what she always wanted.*

Fiona is shown often markedly confused in her environment and fills her conversations with platitudes. She, however, remains composed and does not lose her decorum ("she is a lady"). Most interesting and accurately portrayed is the part when Grant is not sure if she is putting up a charade ("some kind of punishment") by not recognizing him as her husband but then having periods of lucidity. She progresses, stays in bed for weeks, and then has to be moved to another section where the more severely affected people reside ("the second floor"). The movie is based on a short story by Alice Munro.

A film that is one of the most deceptive in its depiction of dementia is the great love story in *The Notebook* (2004) ◁. The film starts with an older couple, James Garner (Duke) and Gena Rowlands (Allie). Allie has advanced Alzheimer's disease, and there are multiple flashbacks to their complicated romance. She does not recognize her children. The children tell Duke to come home, but he wants to be with "his sweetheart." He reads her a story she likes very much but she does not recognize that it is her own life story. ("It is a good story. I heard it before, perhaps more than once?") Suddenly, in a moment of lucidity, all becomes clear, and she remembers everything—but only briefly—and immediately snaps in agitated angry behavior. Other moments of lucidity occur despite more progressive decline. This time she asks "What will happen when I cannot remember anything anymore?" to which he answers, "I'll be here." The film points toward a common theme of caregivers hoping for a single moment when there is full recollection, but it is misleading in suggesting that emotional bonding could lead to such a lucky moment. Terminal lucidity exists, but it is exceptional.

Many films on dementia may not have been seen by the general public, and one paper by Asai discusses ten films from Japanese cinema. This paper emphasizes the difficulty of telling patients they have Alzheimer's and the anger it can cause in spouses. Despair, disbelief, anger toward the spouse, and suicide attempts and care of a severely disabled husband (played by Ken Watanabe) are shown in *Memories of Tomorrow* (2006) ⏴⏴, a popular movie in Japan. It is difficult to see his coping with Alzheimer's any differently than overplaying the frustration faced by early Alzheimer's (his anger is dramatic). The age of onset here is late 40s in a business executive, further adding to its drama.

Memories of Tomorrow has some recognizable themes (dementia in a highly functioning person) and some new ones. It uses early-onset Alzheimer's as a theme—a highly uncommon scenario. The onset of dementia is portrayed in the wife noticing her husband missing an exit while driving and then noticing that he has bought many shampoo bottles—more than needed—which prompts her to seek medical advice.

We see him deteriorating, not being able to find his office and running frantically through Tokyo. We see him unable to find his wife in a restaurant, accusing his wife of infidelity, unable to speak at his daughter's wedding, and eventually retiring in a serene home in the woods. He eventually watches sunsets while being vegetative in a wheelchair. The film moved many viewers in Japan.

Other films have used dementia as a theme, but without further insight. *Firefly Dreams* (2001) is about a self-absorbed teenager taking care of a person with Alzheimer's disease. The Hindi film *Black* (2005) and *I Did Not Kill Gandhi* (2005) have depicted Alzheimer's without much distortion of medical facts. In *U Me Aur Hum* (*You, Me and Us*) (2008) the protagonist is pregnant and suffers from early-onset dementia, but the portrayal is theatrical and does not provide any additional insight.

Several other films have depicted certain aspects of Alzheimer's disease quite well. These include *Iron Lady* (2011), which depicts visual and auditory hallucinations, and more recently the celebrated film *Nebraska* (2013), where the leading character with dementia, Woody (played by Bruce Dern), shows the urge to wander but also shows detachment and he answers many questions about the past with "I don't remember."

A Final Word

Dementia is often accurately depicted in film and usually involves early but not terminal care. In the films discussed here, there is an honest account in *Iris, Song for Martin*, and *Away from Her*, but a fictional account is presented in the much-lauded *The Notebook*. The portrayal often involves disorientation and wandering, but rarely combative behavior. It emphasizes the inability of Alzheimer's patients to recognize themselves, their actions, and their spouses. The fiction films can be seen together with the documentaries discussed in Chapter 5.

Further Reading

Arevalo-Rodriguez I, Pedraza OL, Rodriguez A, et al. Alzheimer's disease dementia guidelines for diagnostic testing: A systematic review. *Am J Alzheimers Dis Other Demen* 2013;28:111–19.

Asai A, Sato Y, Fukuyama M. An ethical and social examination of dementia as depicted in Japanese film. *Med Humanit* 2009;35:39–42.

Balasa M, Gelpi E, Antonell A, et al. Clinical features and APOE genotype of pathologically proven early-onset Alzheimer disease. *Neurology* 2011;76:1720–25.

Garrard P, Maloney LM, Hodges JR, Patterson K. The effects of very early Alzheimer's disease on the characteristics of writing by a renowned author. *Brain* 2005;128:250–60.

Gerritsen DL, Kuin Y, Nijboer J. Dementia in the movies: The clinical picture. *Aging Ment Health* 2014;18:276–80.

Gretton C, Ffytche DH. Art and the brain: A view from dementia. *Int J Geriatr Psychiatry* 2014;29:111–26.

Macip S. Love's memories lost. *The Lancet Neurology* 2007;6:675.

Sadowsky CH, Galvin JE. Guidelines for the management of cognitive and behavioral problems in dementia. *J Am Board Fam Med* 2012;25:350–66.

Segers K. Degenerative dementias and their medical care in the movies. *Alzheimer Dis Assoc Disord* 2007;21:55–59.

PARKINSON'S DISEASE IN FILM

A Late Quartet (2012); starring Christopher Walken, Philip Seymour Hoffman, and Catherine Keener; directed by Yaron Zilberman, written by Yaron Zilberman and Seth Grossman; distributed by Entertainment One.

Rating

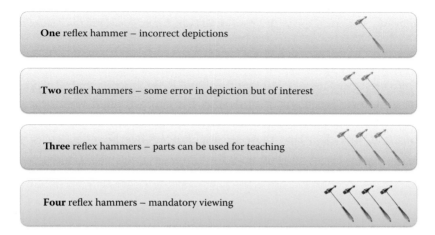

One reflex hammer – incorrect depictions

Two reflex hammers – some error in depiction but of interest

Three reflex hammers – parts can be used for teaching

Four reflex hammers – mandatory viewing

Criticism and Context

How Parkinson's disease over time can affect someone's life and musical ability is the major theme here. The film deals with the consequences of early diagnosis of Parkinson's disease in a closely knit string quartet that is celebrating its 25th anniversary.

The representation of Parkinson's disease in this film is very accurate because the director asked neurologists Stanley Fahn and Lewis Rowland, among others, for advice. Christopher Walken plays Peter, the cellist and founder of this quartet. During a practice session he discovers the inability to move his left hand and fingers well enough to produce a colorful vibrato (oddly enough, primarily a hand-shaking oscillating movement). The female neurologist is played by Madhur Jaffrey, who is compassionate and instructs him to make rapid hand-opening and -closing movements, to stand up and walk a few steps, and to turn around. He shows left-sided hypokinesis, with no instability in arm swing, gait, or balance. The meeting with the neurologist is a notable scene, in particular because Peter is surprised that the diagnosis is a clinical assessment and not a laboratory test with a positive or negative result.

Quotable Lines of Dialogue

A Late Quartet	
Neurologist	*Well, based on the examination that we just ran and the complaints you've described to me, it's my opinion that you are experiencing the early symptoms of Parkinson's disease.*

A Late Quartet	
Patient	*From this… from what we just did, you can tell that?*
Neurologist	*Yes, I am afraid I can; but we should still run a blood test and have the MRI.*
Patient	*Wow.*

The consequences are substantial, and Peter knows that a replacement should be found for him despite his being treated with medication. "I may be able to play one season, but then it will be over." For all of them, it is clear that their season choice—Beethoven's *Late String Quartet Opus 131 in C-Minor*, with its 40 minutes of uninterrupted playing—requires perfectly functioning basal ganglia.

Christopher Walken may be the most ideal actor to play Peter, and he truly shows the appearance of hypokinesis and lack of mimicry. (Playing a subdued and monotonous character is one of Walken's trademarks.) As befits a serious film, it also shows a Parkinson's rehabilitation group (the Brooklyn Parkinson's group, known for dance therapy), where it is emphasized that "in Parkinson's disease everything gets small…everything contracts and closes in," and the goal is to "push those boundaries out." After treatment, Peter has a brief visual hallucination where he sees his late wife (a mezzo-soprano) singing, and there is an episode where he contemplates suicide—all familiar issues in the long-term management of Parkinson's disease.

Suddenly, and much to his surprise, he discovers during a teaching class that he is able to play very well ("the medication is working"), and he rallies his quartet members to practice again. However, while he was resting and taking a break, the supposedly coherent and civilized quartet has fallen apart due to marital problems and flings left and right. The quartet explodes during a practice session in a cathartic. Nevertheless, the quartet reconvenes, and the new season starts. Peter knows that he cannot play the *Presto* fifth movement of Beethoven's late quartet, and he suddenly stops during the first performance, and after a moving speech, introduces a replacement cellist.

The film shows the enormous impact a tiny change in motor function can bring about—common knowledge for all neurologists first diagnosing a neurodegenerative disease. When professional musicians develop Parkinson's disease, it is often career ending and, sadly, early in the process. Inability to quickly switch finger positions could result in loss of tempo, and playing long stretches of music that require close harmonization with other musicians must be quite difficult. While many patients with Parkinson's disease are successfully treated and lead valuable lives, playing complex musical parts not only becomes physically demanding, but memorizing transitions and tremendous attention may not be possible if cognition becomes impaired in later stages. In these situations, successfully treating the movement disorder in tremor-dominant asymmetric Parkinson's disease may not resolve the issue completely. It is also likely much different than treatment of focal dystonia—a disorder commonly found in musicians.

Musicians and composers may have a major illness, just like anyone else, but there is some fascination about how it can affect their creativity. Systemic and neurologic illness have been carefully studied in many classical composers, and a considerable presence of venereal disease has been documented. Parkinson's disease is not well known in famous contemporary musicians or composers. Johnny Cash was diagnosed with Parkinson's disease and then allegedly multiple system atrophy. If the last diagnosis was correct, this may have spared his cognitive abilities and enabled him to even record landmark albums before his final months (i.e., the legendary *American Recordings*). Most rock and roll musicians—with some taking a variety of potentially damaging drugs—seem to have been spared from nigrostriatal injury.

A much less convincing film is *Love & Other Drugs* (2010), in which Anne Hathaway plays a patient (Maggie) with young-onset Parkinson's. Her representation—showing tapping fingers to nonsensically mimic resting tremor—is all we see. She is also seen trying to open a pillbox during a tremor, possibly simulating abnormal finger-eye coordination as an early sign, but again with unusual trembling. In this film, nothing is said about the daily challenges and fatigue. The film shows a self-help meeting of (real) Parkinson's patients, but it is characterized by juvenile jokes. However, there is one key scene where the husband of a patient with advanced Parkinson's disease and asks if he has any advice. Tells Maggie's friend "My advice is to go upstairs, pack up your bags, leave a nice note, and find yourself a healthy woman." In another key scene, Maggie does point out a reasonable list of other diagnoses that have been considered—in her case essential tremor, Wilson's disease, MSA, PSP, obscure dystonia, and surprisingly, neurosyphilis. She also mentions a "scary 6-month brain tumor week", but in the end "it turned out to be old-fashioned Parkinson's disease." The film has some good to say about acceptance of Parkinson's disease, but there is little here that advances the knowledge of living with Parkinson's disease, and much of it is dismissive and contrived.

Early Parkinson's disease (called Stage I in this film and likely referring to the Hoehn and Yahr scale indicating unilateral disease) has other features, typically difficulty with moving (slow walking, hesitance, and difficulty standing up; less mimicry or "poker face"; and less gesticulation with speech). Tremor is at rest when the hand is in a lap, and the voice becomes soft and monotone. Voice and face akinesia occur first, followed by rigidity, gait abnormalities, limb bradykinesia, and finally tremor. In young-onset Parkinson's disease, postural reflexes often remain preserved. None of this is seen in Maggie, even when she is shown to be off medication.

A Final Word

Music and Parkinson's disease are closely connected, generally in a good way. Patients with Parkinson's disease may successfully use musical rhythms for gait initiation, and the enjoyment of music—hearing a favorite musical piece or song—not only may remain present for quite some time, but could potentially also lift them up physically. However, slowing of motor function hampers musicians. During his farewell speech in *A Late Quartet*, Peter explains that he cannot keep up and he cannot play the piece in one uninterrupted session (*attacca*): "It is Beethoven's fault."

Further Reading

Bogousslavsky J, Boller F, eds. *Neurological disorders in famous artists*. Basel: S Karger, 2005.

Ergun U, Bozbas A, Akin U, Inan L. Musical hallucinations and Parkinson disease. *Neurologist* 2009;15:150–52.

Neumayr A. *Music and medicine*. 3-volume set. Lansing, MI: Medi-Ed Press, 1997.

Parashos S, Wichmann R, Melby T. *Navigating life with Parkinson disease*. New York: Oxford University Press, 2012.

Postuma RB, Lang AE, Gagnon JF, Pelletier A, Montplaisir JY. How does parkinsonism start? Prodromal parkinsonism motor changes in idiopathic REM sleep behaviour disorder. *Brain* 2012;135:1860–70.

Schrag A, Ben-Shlomo Y, Brown R, Marsden CD, Quinn N. Young-onset Parkinson's disease revisited—Clinical features, natural history, and mortality. *Mov Disord* 1998;13:885–94.

NEUROGENETICS IN FILM

Lorenzo's Oil (1992); starring Nick Nolte, Susan Sarandon, and Peter Ustinov; directed by Doug Miller, written by George Miller and Nick Enright; Academy Award nominations for best actress (Susan Sarandon) and original screenplay; distributed by Universal Pictures.

Rating

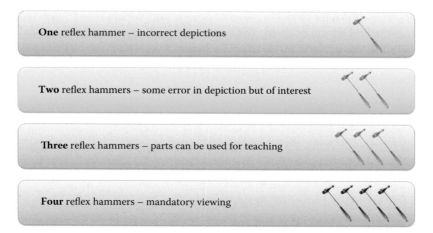

The Cake Eaters (2009); starring Kristen Stewart, Aaron Stanford, Jayce Bartok, Bruce Dern, and Elizabeth Ashley; directed by Mary Stuart Masterson, written by Jayce Bartok; awards at US film festivals—Sedona, Stony Brook, Ashland; distributed by 7-57 Releasing.

Rating

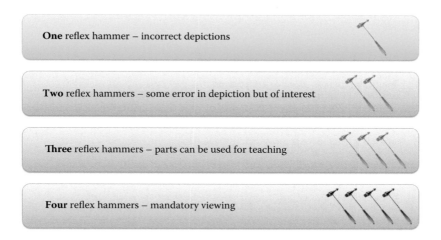

The Madness of King George (1994); starring Nigel Hawthorne, Helen Mirren, Ian Holm, Amanda Donohoe, Rupert Graves, and Rupert Everett; directed by Nicholas Hytner; Academy Award for best art direction (Ken Adams and Carolyn Scott), BAFTA Award for best British film, best actor (Nigel Hawthorne), and best makeup (Lisa Westcott); distributed by Samuel Goldwyn Company.

Rating

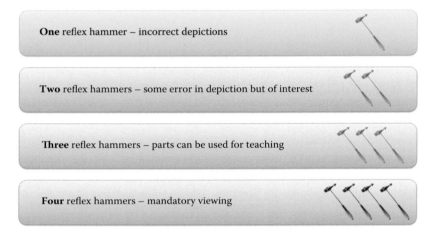

One reflex hammer – incorrect depictions

Two reflex hammers – some error in depiction but of interest

Three reflex hammers – parts can be used for teaching

Four reflex hammers – mandatory viewing

Extraordinary Measures (2010); starring Brendan Fraser, Harrison Ford, and Keri Russell; directed by Tom Vaughan, written by Robert Nelson Jacobs; distributed by CBS Films.

Rating

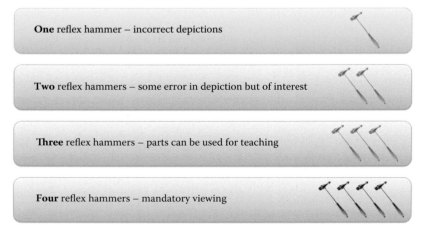

One reflex hammer – incorrect depictions

Two reflex hammers – some error in depiction but of interest

Three reflex hammers – parts can be used for teaching

Four reflex hammers – mandatory viewing

Criticism and Context

Genetics will likely appear more often in film now that the field of neuroge-netics dominates major discoveries and new treatments. In film, neurogenet-ics started in 1992 with *Lorenzo's Oil*, which created such a great controversy as a result of its therapeutic claims that it, perhaps unprecedentedly, prompted editorial comments in the *New England Journal of Medicine* and *The Lancet*.

The film is based on Lorenzo Odone (Figure 3.10). Lorenzo (played, as he ages, by several actors) is a 6-year-old child who becomes irritated easily, develops tantrums, and is diagnosed with adrenoleukodystrophy (ALD). The film starts with teachers pointing out to the parents (Augusto and Michaela Odone, played by Nick Nolte and Susan Sarandon) that Lorenzo has a disturbed behavior and suggests he needs a special aid class, to which his mother replies, "The special aid our son needs will be pro-vided at home."

The visit with the pediatric neurologist, Professor Nikolais (Peter Ustinov impersonating Hugo Moser, after the diagnosis is established), is realistic, and the disorder (with "abnormal very long-chain satu-rated fat" and "they have no enzyme to break it up" and "all we can hope for is to slow the cascade of symptoms") is explained reasonably well, including the genetics. "ALD is passed only through the mother. It goes from mother to son." Myelin is explained as plastic run around electrical wires.

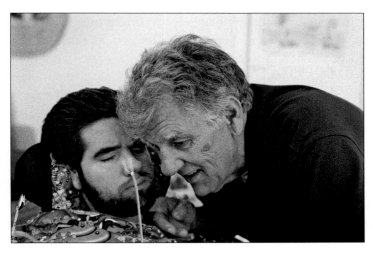

FIGURE 3.10 Lorenzo Odone and his father. (Used with permission of the Myelin Project.)

Quotable Lines of Dialogue

Lorenzo's Oil	
Pediatric neurologist	*It is the cruelest kind of genetic lottery.... No one is to blame.*
Lorenzo's mother	*All these experts working in isolation, each one on its own piece of the jigsaw.*

The parents seek a treatment and there seems to be initial improvement, but the rest of the film shows the boy's decline (with spastic ataxic gait likely shown by a double) to a minimally conscious state. At the end of the film, during the credits, several perfectly healthy-looking children tell the audience they have been on Lorenzo's oil for years.

Adrenoleukodystrophy is a rare X-linked disorder affecting 1 in 20,000 males. At the time of his diagnosis, Lorenzo's parents were told he could live a few years at the most, but he lived until the age of 30 years. The parents desperately tried to find a therapy that could halt the relentless progression. The disorder results in dementia, loss of senses (sight, hearing), and ataxia due to storage of the so-called very-long-chain saturated fatty acids, resulting in demyelination. The accumulation of these lipid chains is a result of impaired degradation through peroxisomal β-oxidation.

In the film, clinical efficacy is suggested using oleic acid (unsaturated short chain) and erucic acid, which are potent competitive inhibitors. This drama of a miracle cure prompted a strong critique by one of the leading experts, Dr. Hugo Moser. Lorenzo's oil may prevent progression in some patients, but mostly when they are asymptomatic. Once the disease is advanced, there is no benefit. The film also dramatizes the parent–physician conflict and inaccurately introduces a scene where the United Leukodystrophy Foundation objects to use of its oil. Rosen summarized the film as portraying "nurses as heartless, physicians as pompous fools, and parent support groups as mindless as a herd of sheep."

Current opinion is divided, but there is some compelling evidence that this oil may prevent the disease from becoming symptomatic. For Lorenzo, the oil did very little, resulting in eventual progression of the disease.

Finding a cure for another devastating neurologic illness is the theme of *Extraordinary Measures*. Brendan Fraser is John Crowley, a biotechnology executive who has three children who are affected by Pompe disease (first described by a female Dutch pathologist in 1932). Pompe disease is a result of a deficiency of the lysosomal enzyme acid alpha-glucosidase, which breaks glycogen links. The film almost immediately confronts the viewer with a child in a motorized wheelchair and another severely paralyzed. Both are tracheostomized and fed through a gastrostomy. Megan's eighth birthday party is the setup of the story. An underlying respiratory infection brings Megan to the ICU, and in an accurately portrayed physician–parent interaction, the physician tells the family there is nothing more that can be done, and she is already past the normal life expectancy (classic Pompe rarely survives the first infantile year). After a successful resuscitation, the parents feel something needs to be done. Contact with an expert, Dr. Stonehill (Harrison Ford)—representing a fictional composite of scientists—leads to discovery of an enzyme that provides a halt to progression.

Quotable Lines of Dialogue

Extraordinary Measures	
Mother to Megan	*I mean, do we just accept our fate and do what we are told by all well-meaning doctors and wait for the worst to happen...or do we fight it?*
John to Dr. Stonehill	*The man is a genius. He is on the verge of a scientific breakthrough.*
Dr. Stonehill	*I am not on the verge of anything.... It is just a theory.... I am just an academic.*

The film is generally neurologically and scientifically accurate, but it remains difficult to have a child "play" a major scoliosis, marked difficulty with breathing, and an absent smile due to facial muscle involvement. (In the movie, Megan smiles all the time.) Since 2006, enzyme replacement therapy for this devastating glycogen-storage disease has resulted in some success in less-affected patients (predominantly in those with normal muscle architecture).

Extraordinary Measures is a carefully crafted film, with excellent representation of physician–parent interaction, the complex science behind the disease, and—less relevant for this book—the funding of research by universities versus the industry. The film is based on the book *The Cure* by Geeta Anand.

The Cake Eaters introduces Friedreich's ataxia—a neurologic disorder for which there is no treatment and that results in progressive ataxia, dysarthria, spasticity, and cardiomyopathy. The disorder is here clearly chosen to add pathos to the life of a teenager afflicted with a neurodegenerative disease. The director contacted several persons with Friedreich's disease and sought input from FARA (Friedreich's Ataxia Research Alliance).

Kristen Stewart plays Georgia, a 15-year-old who falls easily and locks herself up in her home. She displays marked ataxia and slurred speech and walks holding on to a wall in school or is assisted by friends. She refuses a wheelchair when one is offered. None of the common difficulty with fine dexterity is shown. She feels a sense of urgency now that she has been diagnosed, which leads to poor decisions. However, the progression and potential fatality of the cardiac disease is discussed. There is no further neurologic insight or discussion of the consequences of the disease and therefore the film is of little interest to physicians.

Quotable Lines of Dialogue

The Cake Eaters	
Georgia	*I have Friedreich's ataxia.*
Boyfriend	*Is that why you talk drunk?... Are you going to get better?*
Georgia	*This is pretty much as good as it gets until my heart goes out. I wonder when that is going to be.*

The Madness of King George focuses on the agitation and eccentric behavior associated with acute porphyria. The film starts with King George III developing excruciating abdominal pain and then suddenly recovering from what he says was one of his "smart bilious attacks." Attention is focused toward his urine color, which is at one point dark and at another point blue.

Acute porphyria is known to have neuropsychiatric symptoms, although its true spectrum is often misunderstood and exaggerated. Neuropsychiatric manifestations of porphyria—significant confusion, hallucinations, and psychotic breaks—have been reported repeatedly in the literature, but there is very little to support such a connection. However, it is well known that acute porphyria can cause posterior reversible encephalopathy syndrome, which can present as acute confusion, seizures, and a decreased level of consciousness. These symptoms are all reversible after an attack has subsided. Another clear neurologic known manifestation is peripheral motor neuropathy.

Apparently, King George III had four bouts of mental derangement in October 1788, February 1801, January 1804, and October 1810. This incapacity could last six months and resulted in "dementia" and the king's replacement by the Prince of Wales. There has been significant speculation about whether these events can be explained by acute porphyria. Apparently, attending physicians to King George III recorded the unusual colors in his urine, including a blue pigment and blue ring on glass.

The historical arguments against acute porphyria for King George III's spells and attacks are the rarity of the disease, lack of clinical features in his descendants in a disorder that has a high penetrance, the atypical presentation, and the often inaccurate association of psychiatric disorders with acute porphyria. A recent article in *The Lancet* suggested that analysis of hair showed high concentrations of arsenic, a popular medicine in the eighteenth century used as a tonic for treatment of syphilis and skin lesions. Dr. Willis, who portrays an important role in the movie, shows His Majesty being given medication by force. Apparently, the medication given to the king included laudanum as well as zinc, iron, and copper salts. The suggestion is made that arsenic might have exacerbated acute porphyria.

The attack in acute porphyria is associated with increased urinary excretion of porphobilinogen. There is also an increased excretion of aminolevulinate. Many patients have significant abdominal pain, and vomit. Pain may also be in muscles, back, buttocks, and thighs, and the abdominal pain may suggest peritonitis. A significant dysautonomia includes tachycardia and hypertension. These symptoms of heart racing are also mentioned in the film.

A Final Word

Genetic aberrations may lead to rapid disability, and in some, a major neurodegenerative disease. The consequences of these disorders, to the viewer, are understandably important themes and may provide insight. However, in *Lorenzo's Oil* there is an emphasis on curing a complex disease with a relatively simple dietary intervention that may be deceiving. Each of these films is useful for pediatric neurologists and neurogeneticists.

Further Reading

Akst J. A review of *Extraordinary Measures*. *The Scientist Magazine* 2010. http://www.the-scientist.com/?articles.view/articleNo/28726/title/A-review-of-Extraordinary-Measures/ (accessed April 8, 2014).

Arnold WN. King George III's urine and indigo blue. *Lancet* 1996;347:1811–13.

Aubourg P, Adamsbaum C, Lavallard-Rousseau MC, et al. A two-year trial of oleic and erucic acids ("Lorenzo's oil") as treatment for adrenomyeloneuropathy. *N Engl J Med* 1993;329:745–52.

Cox TM, Jack N, Lofthouse S, et al. King George III and porphyria: An elemental hypothesis and investigation. *Lancet* 2005;366:332–35.

Crimlisk HL. The little imitator—porphyria: A neuropsychiatric disorder. *J Neurol Neurosurg Psychiatry* 1997;62:319–28.

Hift RJ, Peters TJ, Meissner PN. A review of the clinical presentation, natural history and inheritance of variegate porphyria: Its implausibility as the source of the "royal malady." *J Clin Pathol* 2012;65:200–5.

Hindmarsh JT. King George III and acute porphyria. *Lancet* 1997;349:364.

Kishnani PS, Beckemeyer AA, Mendelsohn NJ. The new era of Pompe disease: Advances in the detection, understanding of the phenotypic spectrum, pathophysiology, and management. *Am J Med Genet C Semin Med Genet* 2012;160C:1–7.

Koeppen AH. Nikolaus Friedreich and degenerative atrophy of the dorsal columns of the spinal cord. *J Neurochem* 2013;126 Suppl 1:4–10.

Macalpine I, Hunter R. The "insanity" of King George 3d: A classic case of porphyria. *Br Med J (Clin Res Ed)* 1966;1:65–71.

Maramattom BV, Zaldivar RA, Glynn SM, Eggers SD, Wijdicks EFM. Acute intermittent porphyria presenting as a diffuse encephalopathy. *Ann Neurol* 2005;57:581–84.

Moser HW. Lorenzo's oil. *Lancet* 1993;341:544.

Moser HW. Adrenoleukodystrophy: Phenotype, genetics, pathogenesis and therapy. *Brain* 1997;120:1485–1508.

Parkinson MH, Boesch S, Nachbauer W, Mariotti C, Giunti P. Clinical features of Friedreich's ataxia: Classical and atypical phenotypes. *J Neurochem* 2013;126 Suppl 1:103–17.

Rizzo WB. Lorenzo's oil—Hope and disappointment. *N Engl J Med* 1993;329:801–2.

Rosen FS. Pernicious treatment. *Nature* 1993;361:695.

van der Ploeg AT, Clemens PR, Corzo D, et al. A randomized study of alglucosidase alfa in late-onset Pompe's disease. *N Engl J Med* 2010;362:1396–1406.

van der Ploeg AT, Reuser AJ. Pompe's disease. *Lancet* 2008;372:1342–53.

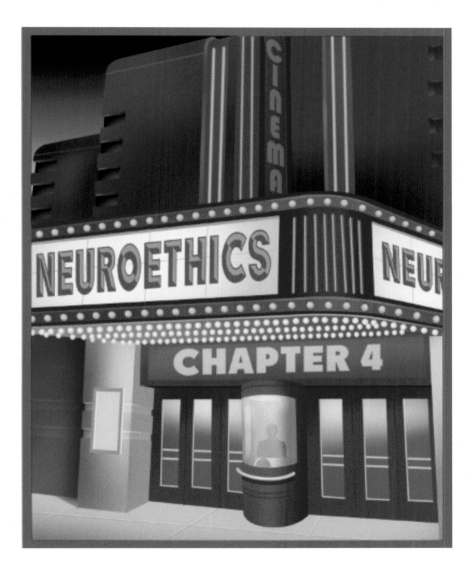

CHAPTER 4

Neuroethics in Film

The only thing worse than your kid dying on you is him wanting to.

The Sea Inside (2004)

INTRODUCING MAIN THEMES

Neurologic disease invites cinematic treatment of commonly encountered bioethical concerns. As expected, the interest of screenwriters is piqued by major topics such as euthanasia in devastating neurologic disease, brain death, and organ donation (and the far more entertaining topic of organ trafficking). Unethical experimentation and lack of informed consent are always of interest and are bound to provoke the audience, and some screenwriters are willing to go an extra mile. In *An Act of Murder* (1948) ⁘ there is a "mercy killing" when a brain tumor causes unbearable pain. In this film, the patient is killed in a car crash caused by her lover in an attempt to end it all. He survives and has to stand trial to argue his motivation, and does so with success. Medical ethics can be largely ignored, and who does not remember Frankie (Clint Eastwood) in *Million Dollar Baby* ⁘ (2004) sneaking into the hospital ward to disconnect a paralyzed ex-boxer from the ventilator? Such scenes get media attention, but we do not know if Hollywood cares about this misrepresentation.

In reality, there are major challenges to be dealt with, and some of it is desperately sad. There is the decision of whether to withdraw care in patients when treatment is considered futile; the decision of patients not to proceed with long-term care; and conflicting situations within families.

There are also sociologic concerns. When to move a family member with advanced dementia to a nursing home has been addressed in feature films. Ethics in film also may involve the compassionate care of neurologic patients.

These bioethical topics are portrayed in many films and touch all specialties, and thus are a potentially rich source of teaching and discussion. The examination of neuroethics in film can be very interesting, and the reason for including it in this book will become abundantly clear when we watch the films discussed in this chapter. Some of them are "mandatory" watching, not necessarily because what is portrayed is right, but more often because it is wrong or highly debatable.

PHYSICIAN-ASSISTED SUICIDE IN FILM

You Don't Know Jack (2010); starring Al Pacino, Danny Huston, Susan Sarandon, and John Goodman; directed by Barry Levinson, written by Adam Mazer; Golden Globe Award and Emmy Award for outstanding lead actor for Al Pacino; distributed by HBO Films.

Rating

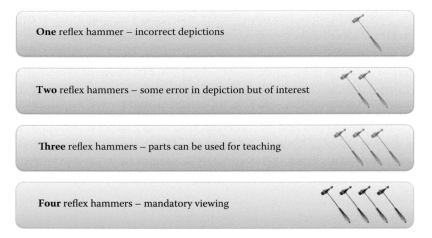

One reflex hammer – incorrect depictions

Two reflex hammers – some error in depiction but of interest

Three reflex hammers – parts can be used for teaching

Four reflex hammers – mandatory viewing

Criticism and Context

The euthanasia movement did not start with Jack Kevorkian. The Euthanasia Society of America was founded in 1938. The initial successes in swaying public opinion were rapidly nullified after the Second World War when euthanasia became associated with the Nazi euthanasia program. The right-to-die movement gained some momentum after the Karen Ann Quinlan and Nancy Cruzan cases of persistent vegetative state, but there has been no substantial change in physician-assisted suicide laws. Despite initiatives in many US states, physician-assisted suicide has only become legal in the states of Oregon, Washington, Montana, and Vermont—with restrictions. Physician-assisted suicide is illegal in most countries, including Canada, Australia, all of Asia, and most European countries, including Germany and France. Jack Kevorkian is a different story.

It has taken some time, but finally Jack Kevorkian—arguably one of the most controversial physicians in the United States—is the subject of a biographical motion picture. Kevorkian is portrayed by Al Pacino (Figure 4.1) in a film directed by the acclaimed director Barry Levinson (*Rain Man*). Because progressive neurologic disease, including nonterminal disabilities such as multiple sclerosis, is a common reason for physician-assisted suicide—at least in Kevorkian's view—this film is highly relevant for neurologists.

Medical organizations have always felt a great unease with Kevorkian's ideas, and this is clearly stated early in the movie. ("I love you, Jack, but most colleagues think you are nuts.") Kevorkian's zeal definitively became a controversy when the *British Medical Journal* in 1996 published an editorial entitled "Jack Kevorkian: A Medical Hero," claiming that he had the "rare heroism to make us all feel uncomfortable."

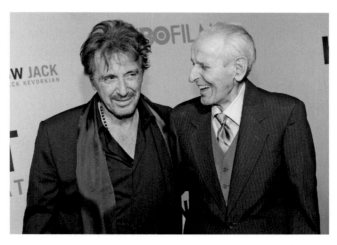

FIGURE 4.1   Al Pacino and Jack Kevorkian. (Used with permission of AP.)

Jack Kevorkian has been admired, ignored, and caricatured. He was a celebrity and was greeted with applause on many talk shows. His infamous Volkswagen minivan—where he assisted patients in their suicide after driving to meet them in remote places—has been for sale on eBay. His macabre artwork shows Nazi symbols and decapitations. One of his paintings has been used as an album cover by the sludge metal band Acid Bath.

The medical side of Jack Kevorkian's story has been well documented. Dr. Kevorkian, a pathologist, claimed to have assisted in over 130 deaths. He was tried in court multiple times and was acquitted multiple times. He built two devices. The first, called the Thanatron (*thanos* = death), was a machine built from scraps that provided a combination of barbiturates, a neuromuscular blocker, and potassium chloride. Later, when his medical license was revoked (and possibly because the necessary drugs could not be easily obtained anymore), he changed to the Mercitron (connoting mercy), consisting simply of a carbon monoxide canister and a mask. However, after he administered a lethal injection to a patient (Thomas Youk, a patient with amyotrophic lateral sclerosis [ALS]) and used the television show *60 Minutes* to broadcast the video of Youk's euthanasia in 1998, he was charged with first-degree murder and delivery of a controlled substance. Kevorkian was in prison for 8 years.

The film portrays the evolution of assisted suicide according to Jack Kevorkian very well, but the viewer should be warned because some clips from the original Kevorkian files show actual patients, intermingled with clips of actors. The film shows patients with Alzheimer's disease, ALS, MS, and spinal cord injury. (The inclusion of neurologic disease is an over-representation based on a review of his cases of euthanasia in Oakland County, Michigan, 1990–1998, which showed that 38% had neurologic disease, 25% had terminal illness, and 35% had pain.)

The movie also shows two patients who were rejected by Kevorkian, suggesting that he had personal criteria for selecting patients. In one patient with Parkinson's disease, he says it is not the right time. In another scene, a paraplegic patient with severe facial scarring—shown after a botched suicide attempt—is diagnosed by Kevorkian as depressed and is told with little compassion, "We cannot help you." The screenwriter here suggests that Kevorkian is not available for all of us in despair. How Kevorkian determines to assist a patient in dying is not addressed. Most disturbing is a scene in which a patient is shown struggling with the mask, after which a plastic hood is placed over his head, eventually requiring two attempts to end his life.

The movie suggests that there has been meticulous documentation of these cases by Kevorkian on index cards, and that he used videotaping to show a noncoerced discussion with the patient. In all depicted scenes, the patient flips a switch to set off an infusion or pulls a paper clip from a section of compressed tubing, allowing the drug or gas to go to the patient. The film clearly shows an operation on a shoestring, and one of his assistants, played by John Goodman, says, "Jack Kevorkian is cheap."

In the movie, Jack Kevorkian proclaims that self-determination is a basic human right and emphasizes his desire to "cause a national debate." He comes up with an unusual comparison: Why is it that mentally competent patients cannot decide whether they want to live or die, while physicians are "starving" comatose patients?

Quotable Lines of Dialogue

You Don't Know Jack	
Jack Kevorkian	*You know they started to do this in Europe already…Holland…never here, we are too puritanical.*
Reporter	*There are those who would say about Dr. Jack Kevorkian: "Right message, wrong messenger."*
Attorney	*And who is the right messenger?*

Susan Sarandon plays Janet Good of the Michigan Hemlock Society, who emphasizes that indignity alone can be a reason for wanting to die. The movie is grim, cold, and sad—feelings that are further amplified throughout the movie as it counts the number of patients, names them, and then shows the dead in black and white.

This movie does not glorify Kevorkian—far from it. It is more about the man than the cause, and alternative options for end-of-life care (i.e., comprehensive palliative care) are not provided. Had the movie been a documentary, we might have been shown such options. Pacino received a well-deserved Emmy and a Golden Globe Award for his depiction of Kevorkian, who he portrayed as a bullheaded, obstinate, and principled person. In the special features on the DVD, Kevorkian himself seemed pleased with the portrayal.

Medical societies have already stated that physicians should not actively end life; instead, they should provide comfort and solace. This is a clear distinction from actively ending life. Justification for physician-assisted suicide is thus problematic in many domains (trust, social implications, reputation, and integrity), but adequate pain relief remains necessary, even if it would lead to very high doses of medication. Palliative care has rapidly become more sophisticated, and "a good death" is often a reachable goal.

Other terms—"physician-assisted dying," "death with dignity," or "aiding dying"—sugarcoat a bigger problem. In states and countries where physician-assisted suicide is allowed, no physician is required to honor the request of a patient and can transfer the care to others if there is personal reluctance or ambivalence. A recent systematic review showed that 0.1% to 3% of all deaths are assisted suicide in European countries and the four US states where it is allowed (Table 4.1). There is an increase in the number of assisted suicides, partly explained by better reporting. Advanced cancer remains the most common considered disease, with ALS and multiple sclerosis much less common, along with spinal cord injury.

TABLE 4.1   Legal Framework in Countries where Assisted Dying Is Legal

Country	Legalization
The Netherlands	Euthanasia law since April 2002: Physician-assisted suicide and euthanasia are not punishable if provided by a physician who has met the requirements of due care. The Netherlands is the only country that allows assisted dying also for minors (12–18 years). Dutch physicians have to report all cases.
Belgium	Euthanasia law since September 2002: Euthanasia is not punishable if provided by a physician who has met the requirements of due care. Physician-assisted suicide is not explicitly regulated in the law, but cases reported to the Belgian Federal Control and Evaluation Commission on Euthanasia are treated the same as euthanasia.
Luxembourg	Law of April 2009 stipulates that doctors who carry out euthanasia and assisted suicides will not face "penal sanctions" or civil lawsuits if the requirements are met.
Switzerland	Under Article 115 of the Swiss Penal Code from 1918, assisting in suicide is only punishable when performed with motives of self-interest.
	Euthanasia is forbidden according to Article 114 in the Penal Code.

Country	Legalization
Switzerland (cont.)	Since 1982, right-to-die organizations assist suicides. Switzerland is the only country that allows assisting in suicide not only for residents but also for foreigners.
United States	
	The Oregon Dignity Act, enacted in October 1997, legalizes physician-assisted suicide but not euthanasia.
	The Washington State Death with Dignity Act, enacted in March 2009, legalizes physician-assisted suicide but not euthanasia.
	The Montana Supreme Court stated in the case *Baxter* in September 2009 that nothing in Montana Supreme Court precedent or Montana statutes indicates that physician aid in dying is against public policy.

Source: Adapted from Steck N, et al. Euthanasia and assisted suicide in selected European countries and US states: Systematic literature review. *Med Care* 2013;51:938–44.

A Final Word

The film unfortunately perpetuates the idea that there is a general lack of end-of-life care in hospitals and that doctors are "cowards." Neurologic disease is overrepresented, and the film suggests that once afflicted, patients lack alternatives other than assisted suicide. After the film—if the portrayal of Jack Kevorkian is accurate—a perversity to the entire story appears. Physicians need to know about Jack Kevorkian and his ways, but then should we not forget him?

Further Reading

Murphy TF. A philosophical obituary: Dr. Jack Kevorkian dead at 83 leaving end of life debate in the US forever changed. *Am J Bioeth* 2011;11:3–6.

Quill TE, Batten MP. *Physician-assisted dying: The case for palliative care and patient choice*. Baltimore: Johns Hopkins University Press, 2004.

Roberts J, Kjellstrand C. Jack Kevorkian: A medical hero. *BMJ* 1996;312:1434.

Roscoe LA, Malphurs JE, Dragovic LJ, Cohen D. Dr. Jack Kevorkian and cases of euthanasia in Oakland County, Michigan, 1990–1998. *N Engl J Med* 2000;343:1735–36.

Steck N, Egger M, Maessen M, Reisch T, Zwahlen M. Euthanasia and assisted suicide in selected European countries and US states: Systematic literature review. *Med Care* 2013;51:938–44.

Wylie H, Nicol N. *You Don't Know Jack*. New York: World Audience, 2011.

SELF-DETERMINATION IN FILM

Whose Life Is It Anyway? (1981); starring Richard Dreyfuss, John Cassavetes, and Christine Lahti; directed by John Badham, written by Reginald Rose and Brian Clark; distributed by Metro-Goldwyn-Mayer.

Rating

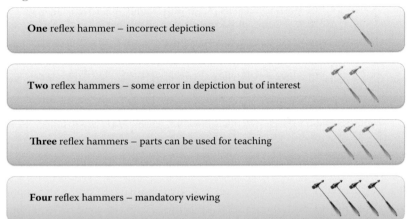

The Sea Inside (*Mar Adentro*) (2004); starring Javier Bardem, Belén Rueda, Lola Dueñas, and Mabel Rivera; directed by Alejandro Amenábar, written by Alejandro Amenábar and Mateo Gil; Academy Award and Golden Globe Award for best foreign language film; distributed by Fine Line Features.

Rating

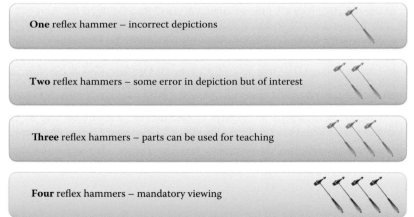

Criticism and Context

In the arts there are numerous examples of patients' self-determination in situations of terminal or disabling illness. These situations can be found in classic fictional literature and theater.

Whose Life Is It Anyway? has been adapted from a play by Brian Clark. (It premiered at the Mermaid Theatre in London and won the Laurence Olivier Award for best new play.) The film accurately depicts the ethical discussion taking place in the early 1980s and considers the competency of sick or injured patients to refuse medical treatment. Ken Harrison (played by Richard Dreyfuss) becomes paralyzed as the result of a severe motor vehicle accident. He also has multiple fractures and, to further add to the drama, as a result of trauma to the kidney, has bilateral nephrectomies requiring permanent dialysis—a strange and unknown surgical indication. He enters the hospital, where Dr. Emerson (chief of medical services, played by the renowned director and actor John Cassavetes) runs into the emergency department, yells at everyone, and slaps Ken in his face, telling him to fight. His condition is discussed with the orthopedic surgeon, who suggests fixing the cervical fracture. Dr. Emerson tells the orthopedic surgeon to keep him alive. After surgery, Ken is seen in the hospital initially joking and making sarcastic remarks. Dr. Emerson tells him he will never walk again or use his arms. Ken, a famous sculptor, decides that this is the end of it; he does not want to stay in the hospital—he wants to go home and die there.

Dr. Emerson is not willing to discuss such an option and orders Valium. When Ken refuses to take the pill, Emerson simply injects it intravenously without Ken's consent. Moreover, he coerces a psychiatrist to find someone ("a staunch Catholic") who would support declaring Ken incompetent. When challenged by one of his colleagues (Christine Lahti, playing Dr. Scott), he says, "Hey, do not give me that right-to-die routine. We're doctors. We are committed to life."

Quotable Lines of Dialogue

Whose Life Is It Anyway?	
Ken	*I decided I do not want to stay alive.*
Dr. Emerson	*You can't decide that.*
Ken	*Why not?*
Dr. Emerson	*Because you are depressed.*

(continued)

Whose Life Is It Anyway? (continued)	
Ken	*Does that surprise you?*
Dr. Emerson	*No, in time you will learn to accept to let us help you.*
Judge	*Do you think you are suffering from depression?*
Ken	*I am completely paralyzed. I think I would be insane if I wasn't depressed.*
Judge	*Yes, but wanting to die must be strong evidence that your mental state has gone far beyond simple depression.*

The film eventually works its way into court where Ken passionately argues for self-determination. Ken calls it an "act of deliberate cruelty" and is outraged that "you have no knowledge of me whatsoever and you have the power to condemn me to a life of torment." Psychiatrists take the stand but are divided on whether this represents a "reactive depression" or a "clinical depression." The judge deliberates and returns, quoting the Karen Ann Quinlan case that decided the preservation of personal right to privacy and right to protest against bodily intrusions, and he even quotes the Saikewicz case which holds that incompetent patients should be afforded the right to refuse life-sustaining treatment (this case is, however, on terminally ill incompetent patients). The judge's final verdict is to allow Ken to leave the hospital if he wishes to do so. Dr. Emerson accepts the court's decision, but asks Ken to stay in the hospital to provide better comfort. "Why?" he asks. "Because you may change your mind!" Ken dies peacefully in the hospital.

The film is useful because of the good back-and-forth arguments of what constitutes patient autonomy. It may even represent the stance of physicians in the 1970s and 1980s who were unwilling to commit to withdrawal of support. The film is well researched legally and medically. Due to its acute observations, it is a landmark in the cinematic depiction of the neuroethics of self-determination.

The Sea Inside has similar themes but is about assisting in dying and is based on the true story of Ramón Sampedro, who died in 1998 at the age of 55 (Figure 4.2). Ramón was left quadriplegic after a diving accident and wrangled for 30 years with the Spanish government to obtain the right to end his life. The decision was made after many years of living with his father, brother, sister-in-law, and nephew, who all participated in his complex care. A daily routine had emerged with the required care, but Ramón, despite all the care, had decided that his life had no dignity. He took on a lawyer who

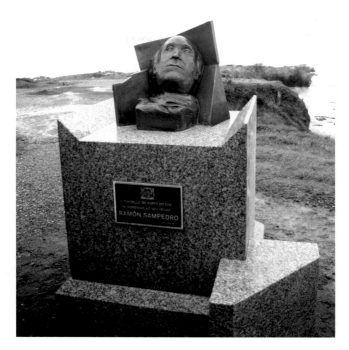

FIGURE 4.2 Sculpture of Ramón Sampedro. The bust was inaugurated in January 2011 and is located at the beach (Playa as Furnas) where Ramón had his accident. (Kindly provided by Manuel G. Teigell.)

specialized in end-of-life care and was an activist, and because she had an inherited neurologic vascular illness, this lawyer "understood" his suffering. His relationship with another woman, Rosa, was different, and she supported continuation of his current existence and the general concept that life is worth living. The film also shows a quadriplegic priest arguing the Catholic position, and their meeting results in a shouting match re-emphasizing the position of each. These contradictions—as expected—are a main focus of this film.

The ending is memorable and shows what happened in real life—a videotape of Ramón drinking from a potassium cyanide solution and dying in front of the camera. This tape was sent to the media and prompted a special commission in the Spanish Senate. Nothing came of it, and physician-assisted suicide or any active withdrawal of support has remained illegal in Spain. The providers of the solution were never found. It has been argued that the media for the first time played an important role in end-of-life discussions—a topic that has largely stayed in academia. Currently, the situation in Spain is that the Constitutional Court has endorsed the right of the individual to deny medical intervention, including medical intervention that could be lifesaving. This was unthinkable in Spain during the first third of the twentieth century, which was dominated by the dictatorship of Franco (1939–1975).

Another assisted withdrawal of care is shown in the provocative film *Million Dollar Baby* (2004) ⁴⁴⁴. The most shocking scene, which has troubled much of the audience, is where Clint Eastwood disconnects the mechanical ventilator of his trainee boxer. Her urge to end her life included forceful biting and injury of her tongue as an act of automutilation. Her loneliness is further emphasized by her family, who ask her to sign her property away to them. She is left alone and cannot fight (literally and emotionally). This final climactic scene created some uproar when the film premiered, but it did not initiate a discussion and did not prevent the film from receiving the Academy Award for best picture. However, most viewers understood that for a visitor to effectively inject a sedative and disconnect the ventilator is highly improbable (even if your name is Clint Eastwood).

The problem addressed in all three of these movies is sudden, devastating, traumatic quadriplegia. Complete cervical transection with apnea usually precludes recovery, but a third of the patients with injuries at the C3 level or lower may recover somewhat. Mortality is around 10% in the first year and doubles in the following decade. The ethical questions in patients with traumatic quadriplegia and ventilator dependency are very difficult. It is highly unusual for a patient with full knowledge of the consequences to ask emphatically to have the ventilator removed. In follow-up interviews at rehabilitation centers, assessments were predominantly positive, with over three-fourths of the patients "glad to be alive." Although many patients express hopelessness and despondency, many also change their mind with the passage of time. Suicide rates are much higher than in a comparable population, but overall are rare (less than 5%). A highly supportive family, marital status, and the availability of resources are important. A productive life is feasible (see *Intouchables* discussed in Chapter 3).

A Final Word

Whether to honor the request to turn off the ventilator requires a comprehensive analysis by an ethics committee. It is difficult to judge whether the patient's request is a rational choice and whether the patient is capable of autonomous choice. The patient should be presented with all relevant facts and rehabilitation options. Postponing the decision is wise, but some patients with a complete transection may continue to forcefully reject any such suggestion. The ventilator can be withdrawn if the patient refuses to reconsider, because any patient may exercise the right to refuse life-sustaining treatment. These decisions are very stressful to caregivers, who may disagree with the decision, and they should seek support. It is well established that physicians—in their own personal judgment—are too pessimistic about "quality of life" for these patients, particularly when there is ventilator dependency. When surviving patients are asked, they rate their quality of life as good and even excellent, and they express a gratitude for being alive.

Further Reading

Annas GJ. Reconciling Quinlan and Saikewicz: Decision making for the terminally ill incompetent. *Am J Law Med* 1979;4:367–96.

Charlifue S, Apple D, Burns SP, et al. Mechanical ventilation, health, and quality of life following spinal cord injury. *Arch Physical Med Rehab* 2011;92:457–63.

Middleton JW, Dayton A, Walsh J, et al. Life expectancy after spinal cord injury: A 50-year study. *Spinal Cord* 2012;50:803–11.

Simón-Lorda P, Barrio-Cantalejo IM. End-of-life healthcare decisions, ethics and law: The debate in Spain. *Eur J Health Law* 2012;19:355–65.

Swartz M. The patient who refuses medical treatment: A dilemma for hospitals and physicians. *Am J Law Med* 1985;11:147–94.

Whalley Hammell K. Quality of life after spinal cord injury: A meta-synthesis of qualitative findings. *Spinal Cord* 2007;45:124–39.

WITHDRAWAL OF SUPPORT IN FILM

The Descendants (2011); starring George Clooney, Shailene Woodley, Beau Bridges, Judy Greer, Matthew Lillard, and Robert Forster; written and directed by Alexander Payne, screenplay by Alexander Payne, Nat Faxon, and Jim Rash; Academy Award for best writing/adapted screenplay and Golden Globe Award for best actor (George Clooney) among many other awards; distributed by Fox Searchlight Pictures.

Rating

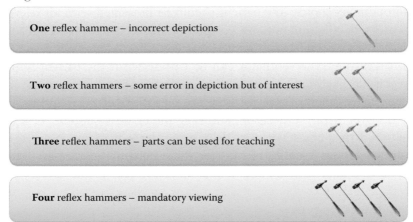

One reflex hammer – incorrect depictions

Two reflex hammers – some error in depiction but of interest

Three reflex hammers – parts can be used for teaching

Four reflex hammers – mandatory viewing

Criticism and Context

The Descendants has many plot elements and is multilayered, but in essence, the premise is quite simple: this is a film about withdrawal of care in a futile situation. The film concentrates on all aspects of withdrawal of support in a patient with a major catastrophic head injury. Matt King (George Clooney) is an attorney in Honolulu who is suddenly faced with his wife, Elizabeth (Patricia Hastie) hospitalized in a coma as a result of a boating accident. She tragically, throughout the film, is shown comatose, and she is one of the best cinematic representations of prolonged coma (Chapter 3). In one of the opening scenes, we see Matt walking into the Queen's Medical Center in Honolulu thinking that she will wake up, they will talk about their marriage, and he will buy her everything she wants. He is certain that he will rediscover their lost love and that they can be close again like in their early days. However, after his discussion with Dr. Johnson, it becomes rapidly apparent that she has no chance of waking up, and her condition is permanent. Matt ignores this conversation with the neurologist, and when his family inquires about her state, he simply says, "Hope for the best and keep the vital organs working."

Quotable Lines of Dialogue

The Descendants	
Dr. Johnson	*I wish I had better news, Matthew, but Dr. Chun and Dr. Mueller agree that her condition is deteriorating. She has no eye movement, no pupillary responses. She has no brainstem reflexes whatsoever. I mean, the machine can keep her alive; but her quality of life would be so poor, basically the way she is now.*

He has a serious and much different conversation with his daughter. In a heartbreaking moment, he tells her he must let Elizabeth go because her living will stipulates it. He tells her they were both very clear about that, should anything happen to either of them. Then, out of the blue, his daughter tells him that his wife had an affair. This is followed by a remarkable scene showing a tremendous unloading of stress. Matt—getting more upset upon hearing that his other family members were also aware of Elizabeth's extramarital relationship—projects his anger. He tells them that what they are doing to Elizabeth—trying to care for her in the hospital—makes no sense. ("You are putting lipstick on a corpse.")

Matt also discusses the advance directive with his father-in-law, who looks at it and says, "It's like reading Korean…jibber jabber." Matt suggests walking through it with him, but his father-in-law tells him he knows exactly what the situation is, and he wants to honor his daughter's wishes. Although there is a resolution within the family and appreciation of Elizabeth's wishes to not be kept in such a state, the film captures the family stressors and fragility during such circumstances very well. It quickly becomes a quietly devastating film.

Elizabeth is in a persistent vegetative state, and great effort has been made to make her look exactly as these patients are. Her sunken facial expression, lack of any mimicry, and with no resemblance to her glamourous photos displayed next to her bed is a stark reminder of what such a condition entails. There is great attention to detail in this film. Observant physicians will note that with every new scene, the writing board in her room changes from "weaning" to "DNR" to "no plan for the day" as she transitions to palliative care.

The film is extraordinarily sensitive in showing the family coming to terms with this catastrophe. There is a poignant break in tension and a tender scene in which Matt says goodbye to his wife followed by scattering her ashes in the ocean off Waikiki. There are very few films that are as frank about withdrawal of care in a futile situation as this one.

Another film that touches on withdrawal of support is *Steel Magnolias* (1998) ✍. Shelby (Julia Roberts), who has type I diabetes, successfully delivers a baby, but several months later she develops kidney failure and starts dialysis. Shelby is found unconscious (through a window we overhear that her coma might be irreversible). There is no explanation of the cause of coma, and when she does not awaken, the ventilator is removed. The scene shows the immediate presence of a bradycardia and arrest without showing the patient. The husband is seen signing a form before withdrawal, another highly unusual procedure (and often in film confused with signing a consent form).

How do these films reflect real-life situations? Advance directives, used in many countries, are legal documents in which the patient has determined what actions should be taken in the event that they are no longer able to make decisions due to illness or incapacity. The documents can come in many forms. Some designate that a power of attorney may make decisions about the patient; others, such as a living will, leave instructions for treatment. Surrogate decision makers may be legally established as a durable power of attorney and are usually members of the patient's family. These advance directives typically specify when there is care in a terminal condition, and these living wills have been clearly written in order not to prolong care in the setting of futility. Physicians will review advance directives, and they need to be addressed with the patient and family members.

In a persistently comatose patient who is unable to make decisions, and never will, a surrogate (mostly spouse) has a major role. The decision to be made is based on the patient's best interests and, as expected, is dependent on the benefits of treatment versus the burdens of treatment. A family that wants to continue aggressive care in a severely brain-injured patient with additional significant other medical concerns should understand there will be a long road of complications. Treatment required with each of these complications may be reassessed.

A do-not-resuscitate (DNR) order is part of a decision that can be put forward in a living will. Many hospitals require that resuscitation orders be addressed upon admission. Families typically request full resuscitative measures upon admission, but they often ask for a DNR status after seeing no progress in care. DNR status may also come into play when physicians see no improvement despite aggressive measures to reverse the condition, or when there is simply a clinical situation that is overwhelmingly bad.

A Final Word

Who would have thought that a feature film would address such major bioethical topics? Virtually all major ethical and social issues are depicted in *The Descendants*. The stress of families waiting for closure, trying to reach consensus among family members, and the futility of critical care under certain circumstances can all be seen in this film. For the viewer it provides an opportunity to discuss one's own values and perceptions.

The issue of advance directives is fairly more recent, and therefore this major neuroethical issue is not often found in film. "Doctor knows best," the "fighting doctor," and the doctor who "never gives up" is what screenwriters were accustomed to presenting. In the real world, there has been a major change in the structure of end-of-life care, and *The Descendants* is a good way to start to examine this.

Further Reading

Foster C. Putting dignity to work. *Lancet* 2012;379:2044–45.

Gerstel E, Engelberg RA, Koepsell T, Curtis JR. Duration of withdrawal of life support in the intensive care unit and association with family satisfaction. *Am J Respir Crit Care Med* 2008;178:798–804.

Lanken PN, Terry PB, Delisser HM, et al. An official American Thoracic Society clinical policy statement: Palliative care for patients with respiratory diseases and critical illnesses. *Am J Respir Crit Care Med* 2008;177:912–27.

Mehta S. The intensive care unit continuum of care: Easing death. *Crit Care Med* 2012;40:700–1.

Truog RD, Cist AF, Brackett SE, et al. Recommendations for end-of-life care in the intensive care unit: The Ethics Committee of the Society of Critical Care Medicine. *Crit Care Med* 2001;29:2332–48.

FAMILY CONFLICTS ON LEVEL OF CARE IN FILM

Critical Care (1997); starring James Spader, Kyra Sedgwick, Helen Mirren, Anne Bancroft, and Albert Brooks; directed by Sidney Lumet, written by Richard Dooling and Steven Schwartz; distributed by Media Works.

Rating

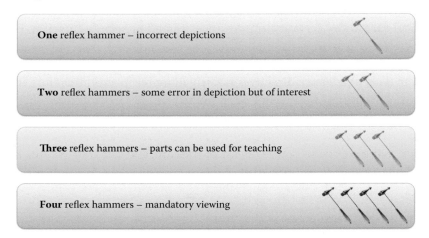

One reflex hammer – incorrect depictions

Two reflex hammers – some error in depiction but of interest

Three reflex hammers – parts can be used for teaching

Four reflex hammers – mandatory viewing

Criticism and Context

Conflicts between family members are very well depicted in this comedy. Although there are exaggerations, the film clearly highlights a common occurrence in intensive care units (ICUs) with families who conflict with each other on what the best level of care might be.

Critical Care starts with introducing a new ICU (with futuristic blue lights and antidecubitus mattresses that look like pool floats) with one of the doctors, Dr. Ernst (James Spader), taking care of several patients. One elderly patient is in a persistent vegetative state after a cardiac arrest. The patient, on a respirator, has been recently moved to the critical care unit. ("Why was daddy moved to this floor?" "He was getting excellent care on the eighth floor, but this is the newest ICU facility.") Connie (played by Margo Martindale) is his half-sister, who wants his life prolonged as long as possible; but Felicia (Kyra Sedgwick) cannot stand it any longer. The movie is a satire on prolonging care and its financial consequences, but even more so on family conflicts. Connie is convinced that he responds ("One squeeze is yes; two squeezes is no. You tell me that is some kind of a seizure?"). She knows because she has been coming to this hospital every single day. She gets angry at the physician ("My father is not terminally ill; he is convalescing"), accusatory ("For the rest of you it is all sneers and laughter"), and paranoid ("I heard nurses and technicians laughing and telling jokes...as if he wasn't a living person in the room"). She also is concerned that her other sister might be doing something to him when they are not around ("I'd watch myself around her"). The film eventually turns into a conflict about inheritance after the patient dies, and it introduces a commonly perceived myth—withdrawal from care to get the inheritance.

How does this translate to real-life ICU practices? There are families of comatose patients who would want to pursue any possible option, who don't recognize the seriousness of the situation, and who often believe that withholding intensive care is a poor decision no matter what. In their minds, every individual should be given the maximum chance, and they cannot comprehend that the physician does not think the same. This film clearly shows a realistic example of such a conflict and is worthwhile as a teachable clip in lectures. In this film, Connie continuously cites the Bible and biblical figures to make her point. The puzzlement of the physician is equally well portrayed here when he is overwhelmed with biblical citations. Religious influence—the "our faith lets us continue on" argument—is prevalent in these situations, emphasizing that life always has value, even if there is suffering. On balance, physicians respect all faiths, and their task in this respect is to say words of comfort and express understanding.

Quotable Lines of Dialogue

Critical Care	
Dr. Ernst	*You wanted to see me?*
Connie	*Oh, yes, I know… if you and my sister were discussing my father's care?*
Dr. Ernst	*Her only concern is that your father's suffering not be prolonged.*
Connie	*I'd watch myself around her. My sister is Delilah, Dr. Ernst. My sister is Salome and Jezebel.*
Dr. Ernst	*Really?*
Connie	*Since my sister does not believe my father should be receiving life support, I don't think it's appropriate to allow her to be alone with him.*

Family conflicts are a significant threat, not only to quality of care, but also to what needs to be a cordial relationship between the treating physicians and concerned family members. Conflicts may also be present within the family structure, as this film so clearly demonstrates. Different opinions may result in the inability to make important decisions for the patient, and in the midst of this conflict, the wishes of the patient may be sidetracked by a combination of trivialities (such as creating irritation with nurses or residents). From a family point of view, conflicts are often related to ineffective communication, professional staff behaviors that include disrespectful or dismissive attitudes, and the perception that there is a time pressure about the decision to stop critical care. Some families do not accept the limits of medicine. Some simply cannot make the decision to stop, even when physicians suggest to curtail care. This may cause a powerful defensive stance of the family that can lead to continuous requests for treatment.

More than anything else, dispute resolution should start with a reappraisal of what caused the conflict. First, a physician with significant communication skills is needed to help all healthcare workers to participate in a family conference. There should be clear reassurance to the family that the patient's cultural attitudes and values are appreciated. Barriers to communication should be identified and improvements should be suggested. Resolution of conflicts can only come with an inordinate amount of time spent with the family explaining the plan and expectations. The consequences of a conflict are not only the safety and quality of care for the patient, but also the progressive mistrust, dissatisfaction, burnout, misunderstanding with staff, and increased healthcare expenditures due to the increased length of stay.

A Final Word

Decisions about care in critically ill patients have rarely been used as a plot. *Critical Care* should be contrasted with *The Descendants*, where decisions are clear and there is resolution and closure. When seen in its totality, this film has many absurdities. It addresses the costs of health care, makes fun of hospital administrators (in a brilliant role of Albert Brooks as Dr. Butz), and suggests that continuation of care in a young, well-insured patient is financially beneficial. One dialyzed patient with vivid hallucinations is fully cared for because the hospital can profit from transplanting kidneys. Dr. Butz also posits that discussions of feeding tubes in the terminally ill are nonexistent. ("You think just because someone's going to die soon, we don't need to feed them? I've news for you! We're all gonna die! So why should any of us eat?") When care of the comatose patient is questioned, he counters, "Where have you been all your life?... It is called revenue."

Although it is humorous, it has provided the audience with a complex topic—family conflict on de-escalation of care when care seems futile. There are a lot of dark remarks, and misperceptions of health care are exposed.

Further Reading

Bloche MG. Managing conflict at the end of life. *N Engl J Med* 2005;352:2371–73.

Boyd EA, Lo B, Evans LR, et al. "It's not just what the doctor tells me": Factors that influence surrogate decision-makers' perceptions of prognosis. *Crit Care Med* 2010;38:1270–75.

Fassier T, Azoulay E. Conflicts and communication gaps in the intensive care unit. *Curr Opin Crit Care* 2010;16:654–65.

Luce JM. A history of resolving conflicts over end-of-life care in intensive care units in the United States. *Crit Care Med* 2010;38:1623–29.

Studdert DM, Mello MM, Burns JP, et al. Conflict in the care of patients with pro-longed stay in the ICU: Types, sources, and predictors. *Intensive Care Med* 2003;29:1489–97.

White DB, Pope TM. The courts, futility, and the ends of medicine. *Jama* 2012;307:151–52.

BRAIN DEATH AND ORGAN DONATION IN FILM

All About My Mother (1999); starring Cecilia Roth, Marisa Paredes, Antonia San Juan, and Candela Peña; written and directed by Pedro Almodóvar; Academy Award and Golden Globe Award for best foreign language film, Goya Award for best actress (Cecilia Roth), for best film, best screenplay, and best director (Pedro Almodóvar), and best supporting actress (Candela Peña); distributed by Sony Pictures Classics.

Rating

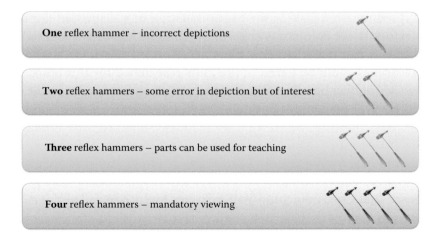

One reflex hammer – incorrect depictions

Two reflex hammers – some error in depiction but of interest

Three reflex hammers – parts can be used for teaching

Four reflex hammers – mandatory viewing

21 Grams (2003); starring Sean Penn, Naomi Watts, and Benicio Del Toro; directed by Alejandro González Iñárritu, written by Guillermo Arriaga; Venice Film Festival Award for best actor (Sean Penn); distributed by Focus Features.

Rating

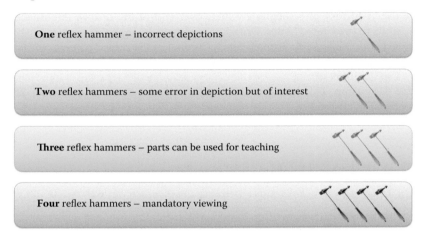

One reflex hammer – incorrect depictions

Two reflex hammers – some error in depiction but of interest

Three reflex hammers – parts can be used for teaching

Four reflex hammers – mandatory viewing

Criticism and Context

Organ donation after a catastrophic neurologic injury is mostly neurologic and neurosurgical terrain. It therefore qualifies as a topic for this book. Many neurologists, when watching these hospital scenes, would feel a familiarity with the cause (severe traumatic brain injury) and the discussion (asking for organ donation in a distressed family). Neurologists are commonly involved with brain death determination and thus organ donation. Few films have tackled this topic, and only single scenes could be found in the films researched for this book. *All About My Mother* has one of the most accurate scenes of organ donation, but there are some important quibbles. The film starts with a "simulation scene" showing the training of organ transplant coordinators. The main character, Manuela (Cecilia Roth), is one of the coordinators. The simulation shows a compassionate discussion on how to obtain consent for organ donation. There is also a very unusual confusion (the proxy believes that organ donation will help her loved one rather than the other way around). Then, in a sudden plot twist, simulation becomes reality when Manuela's son gets hit by a car and is pronounced brain dead. Now she is seen sitting in a cold, gray hallway of the hospital and is approached by two physicians who tell her that the EEG confirms what they already know. Thereafter she is seen signing a consent form. "We have to make decisions immediately," the physician tells her. Her son is then rushed into the operating room, and we see a phone call to the recipient (who displays the stress and confusion of a middle-of-the-night phone call when summoned to come to the hospital). The next scene shows Manuela hiding behind a pillar while watching the recipient come out of the hospital. She admits to a colleague that she has looked up the medical records and found her son's recipient. The rest of the film has little to do with this event, and she moves out of Madrid.

21 Grams is about organ donation and a new life after heart transplantation. Paul (Sean Penn) has terminal heart disease and is awaiting a heart transplant. The key scene is where Cristina (Naomi Watts) is called to the hospital after she receives a phone call that her husband and both daughters were hit by a car. Subsequently, Cristina is seen waiting in the hospital room. The discussions again are taking place in cold concrete waiting rooms. Two physicians approach Cristina and tell her, "Your husband suffered multiple skull fractures. We had to remove blood clots from around his brain.... We are concerned that he's showing low brain activity." The next scene in the hospital shows her discussing organ donation with an organ donor coordinator, and the discussion is compassionate and real.

Quotable Lines of Dialogue

21 Grams	
Transplant coordinator	*As you know, the doctors did everything they could to save your husband's life, but he has shown no brain activity. We're here to help you with some of the final decisions that need to be made. We have a patient who is gravely ill. I am here to give you some information on organ donation. Are you willing for your husband to donate his heart?*
Sister	*Can we discuss this another time?*
Transplant coordinator	*I'm afraid not. I can give you time to discuss it, but this is a decision that needs to be made soon.*

Mary and Paul are also called (again in the middle of the night) to tell them to rush to the hospital because a heart is waiting for him. Now both the recipient and donor family are in the hospital, and this leads to a remarkable scene. Mary is sitting in the waiting room and sees Cristina and family passing by her, walking with the donor's belongings. This is a highly unlikely scenario and cannot occur. In our experience, families leave the hospital long before organs are recovered, and the only instance I am aware of is when the recipients noted the arrival of the transplant surgeon.

Paul is then seen after heart transplantation. ("I have a question for you. Whose heart do I have?") The physician appropriately says he cannot tell, but one of the nurses suggests he write an anonymous letter through the donor association. This is correctly portrayed, as transplant recipients can express gratitude through anonymous correspondence, but confidentiality is maintained. It is a commonly asked question, and organ transplant organizations have clear policies. (See the United Network for Organ Sharing website, www.unos.org.) However, Paul is not so happy with this policy and hires a private investigator, who provides him with medical details (having copies of the hospital record) and the actual address of the donor's wife, Cristina. How the private investigator got this material is not shown but implies that a private investigator may have found a healthcare worker with access—another highly unusual scenario. I accept that it is necessary for the story line, but we should assume that throughout the world, hospital staff maintain patient privacy at all times. (Slipups are not impossible, though.)

Upon reviewing other recent films, it becomes clear that organ donation speaks to the imagination of screenwriters through the controversial topic of organ trafficking. Other major themes are "redemption" and "compassion," but mostly with absurd (though highly entertaining) plots (Table 4.2). Notable examples are *John Q* (2002), where John Quincy Archibald (Denzel Washington) hears that his insurance will not cover his son's heart transplant. In his desperation, he takes the hospital's emergency room hostage and demands that physicians perform the transplant. (He is even willing to kill himself so that he can donate his heart, but there is a twist.) *Never Let Me Go* (2010) is a fantastical plot on children purely prepared as organ donors. *Coma* (1973) is about organ trafficking. *Return to Me* (2000) suggests that the recipient may also inherit the donor's personality traits.

There is no lack of imaginary scenarios. The most macabre scene is in *Monty Python's The Meaning of Life* (1983). A man opens the front door and sees two medics (one played by John Cleese) in white coats: "Hello, can we have your liver?" After it is explained to the man what a liver is,

TABLE 4.2   Recent Films that Feature Organ Donation

Movie	Type	Theme
Never Let Me Go (2010)	Science fiction	Children raised to be organ donors
Repo Men (2010)	Science fiction	Recipient will lose artificial organ if not paid in time
The Island (2005)	Science fiction	People killed for organ donation
John Q (2002)	Thriller	Hospital emergency department held hostage by a father desperate to get his son's name on the list for a heart transplant
Return to Me (2000)	Romance	Transplanted organ can transplant feelings of the donor
Dirty Pretty Things (2002)	Thriller	Organ trafficking
Seven Pounds (2008)	Thriller	Suicide in order to donate organs

he says, "I know what it is. I am using it." He is cornered and his wallet is ripped out of his pocket. "What is this, then?" asks the medic. "A liver donor's card," he answers. The medic retorts, "Need we say more?" The man continues to protest, but the medics proceed with putting a knife in his abdomen, harvesting his liver, and ripping out all the other organs in a big bloody mess. His wife enters the room and asks, "Is this because he took out one of those silly cards?" and adds, "Typical of him.... He goes down to the public library, he sees a few signs up, and comes home all full of good intentions."

In transplantation ethics, a so-called dead donor rule exists that stipulates that when organs that sustain life are removed, the patient must be dead first, and not be killed by removal of those organs. The Monty Python spoof seems to suggest that once you are a registered donor, you should beware of your organs.

A Final Word

The ethics of organ donation are all over the place in film. This may not be surprising, and who would not want to see a good thriller concerning unethical physician behavior, donor–recipient contact, fighting for an organ for a loved one, and the (unfortunately real) practice of organ trafficking? How these plots influence the moviegoer's view on organ donation is not known, and I am not certain whether it is negligible, potentially damaging, or somewhere in between.

Further Reading

Goetzinger AM, Blumenthal JA, O'Hayer CV, et al. Stress and coping in care-givers of patients awaiting solid organ transplantation. *Clin Transplant* 2012;26:97–104.

Miyazaki ET, Dos Santos R, Jr., Miyazaki MC, et al. Patients on the waiting list for liver transplantation: Caregiver burden and stress. *Liver Transpl* 2010;16:1164–68.

Siminoff LA, Agyemang AA, Traino HM. Consent to organ donation: A review. *Prog Transplant* 2013;23:99–104.

INSTITUTIONALIZING IN FILM

The Savages (2007); starring Laura Linney, Philip Seymour Hoffman, and Philip Bosco; written and directed by Tamara Jenkins; Independent Spirit Award for best male lead and best screenplay; distributed by Fox Searchlight.

Rating

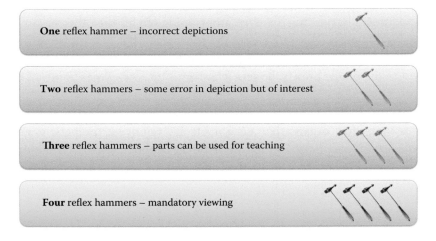

One reflex hammer – incorrect depictions

Two reflex hammers – some error in depiction but of interest

Three reflex hammers – parts can be used for teaching

Four reflex hammers – mandatory viewing

Fred Won't Move Out (2012); starring Elliott Gould, Fred Melamed, Stephanie Roth Haberle, and Judith Roberts; written and directed by Richard Ledes; distributed by Rainwater Films, Ltd.

Rating

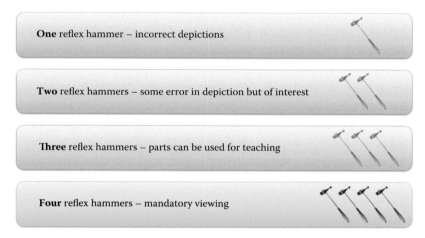

One reflex hammer – incorrect depictions

Two reflex hammers – some error in depiction but of interest

Three reflex hammers – parts can be used for teaching

Four reflex hammers – mandatory viewing

Criticism and Context

The traditional thinking has always been that the elderly cope best when integrated into their own environment. However, after the diagnosis of Alzheimer's disease, the chance of nursing home placement increases rapidly from 20% after 1 year to 50% after 5 years, and over 90% after 8 years. This is substantially higher than in elderly patients without dementia (by comparison 5%–10%). Caregivers' burden is a major factor. In the United States, there are over 9 million people caring for relatives with dementia.

The Savages is one of the more profound films dealing with children facing decisions to place a parent with dementia in a nursing home, often labeled with the deplorable term *institutionalization*. Jon and Wendy (played admirably by the late Philip Seymour Hoffman and Laura Linney) live their own lives, and their father (who has been abusive to them in the past) resides in a well-known senior living community in Arizona (Sun City). Their father, Lenny (played by Philip Bosco), is in a nonmarital arrangement, but then his girlfriend dies. He has to leave because he has no right to use or inherit any of her property. He is rapidly dementing, requiring assistance. The children have been estranged, and they realize it when they visit his home. ("Did you see there were no pictures of us?")

Jon and Wendy see no other way than to move their father to a nursing home, a move that becomes a certainty after Lenny smears feces on the wall and is admitted to the hospital for agitation. Now in the hospital, they find him in restraints and confused ("They have me hogtied for 2 days."), and he accuses his children for not being there when all this happened. ("I know who you are…the late ones.") Both children are now faced with a difficult situation and are frankly overwhelmed by the choice of how to handle this situation properly. The neurologist—who thinks Lenny has Parkinson's disease and not dementia because he does not see any strokes on MRI—does not help either with clarifying the situation.

Jon and Wendy are shown struggling to find a good nursing home, and Lenny is admitted to a drab place. (When Wendy asks Jon, "Do they smell?" Jon answers, "They all smell.") Wendy cleans out Lenny's house, finding cluttered closets, old-man clothes, useless memorabilia, and even an 8-track cartridge—but more importantly, unseen photos of their youth. These photos remind Wendy of a better time, but Jon remains sarcastic and wants nothing to do with it.

In the nursing home, Lenny is seen with a shuffling walk and is mostly agitated and disoriented. The tactless nursing home staff want to know what to do when he dies—burial or cremation. The children are now suddenly forced to discuss these sensitive matters. In a key comic-dramatic scene, the children ask Lenny what he would want to do in case "something happens." When Lenny looks nonplussed, Jon adds, "If you would be in a coma, would you want to be on a ventilator?" Lenny is flabbergasted ("What kind of question is that?") but commits to agreeing to let them "unplug" him. When Jon asks him, "Then what?" he yells, "You bury me!" Indeed, in reality, setting foot into such a facility is overwhelming for family members often being rushed through the admission process and stacks of paperwork.

Wendy tries to find a better nursing home, but Jon is not interested, knowing that none of this matters if Lenny does not know where he is. The effort to find a better nursing home is actually an attempt to make themselves feel better and is not directed at Lenny's needs.

Quotable Lines of Dialogue

The Savages	
Jon	*Do not make me out to be the evil brother putting away our father against your will. We are doing this together, right?*
Jon	*It is not about dad; it is about your guilt…that is what these places prey upon; and all this wellness propaganda and landscaping is just to obscure the miserable fact that people are dying.*

As a result of this experience, both Jon and Wendy relive some old painful memories, although we do not know what really has happened. In the end Lenny dies, but not much changes, and they go on with their lives, perhaps changed, perhaps not.

Fred Won't Move Out is also highly suitable for showing the socioeconomic effects of dementia on an elderly couple. The film is based on a personal memoir and was shot in the house of the director's parents. This is as close as a scripted film can get to a documentary about the troubles with senile parents.

Fred Won't Move Out starts with children visiting their parents (Susan and Fred, Figure 4.3). In the car, it becomes rapidly clear where the problems are: "The thing is, when he is up there by himself, we have no idea what medication he is taking or how much. We don't know if he is taking her medication…. I agree it is totally nuts."

Victoria (called "Queen Victoria" by Fred) is a caretaker from Ghana played by Mfoniso Udofia. The morning scene shows both physically in need. Fred is barely coming off the stairs and Susan is afraid to even sit down. "Good morning, Susan," Fred says. "Whoop-de-doo" is Susan's answer. Susan is more affected than Fred. Music therapy is performed with a piano player, and all are singing Susan's favorite tunes. Susan, who has been nearly catatonic, changes dramatically, smiles, and enthusiastically sings and laughs. Fred says, "It makes her happy; and when she's happy, it makes it much better for all of us."

Their children—Bob (Fred Melamed) and Carol (Stephanie Roth Haberle)—are trying to find a solution after an unclear medical event that suggests something serious could happen with their parents. Both soon also find out that the caretaker is overwhelmed, and that this situation cannot go on. Victoria tries to do the main errands but also wants to keep Fred as active and participatory as possible. When the children find out he has not done his taxes and they confront him, he says, "I do not owe anything."

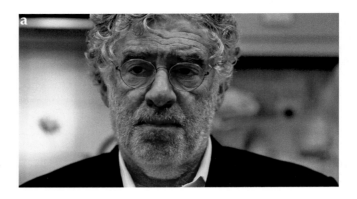

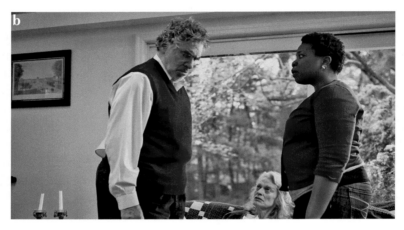

FIGURE 4.3 Scenes in *Fred Won't Move Out*. (a) Fred, played by Elliot Gould; (b) Fred confronted by Victoria, played by Mfoniso Udofia. Susan, played by Judith Roberts, is sitting on the couch. (Used with permission of Richard Ledes.)

In a civil discussion, the children are trying hard to get Fred to agree to move out of his wonderful lake house, and Bob suggests that they are going to live "like in a dorm." That seems agreeable to Susan but not to Fred, and he responds grumpily, not seeing the point of going elsewhere. ("I am not going.")

A tranquil scene shows both children walking through the lot and reminiscing about the past. The film's cutaway scenes show Fred and Susan's house with its fantastic foliage, flowerbeds, and a majestic lake view. We see a seasoned house in all its glory, but with the addition of stacks of medication lined up on the cabinets, the inevitability of growing old also shows.

Well timed in the narrative, Bob tells a wonderful myth of the gods. He tells his children that the gods Zeus and Hermes were looking for disappearing hospitality among the Greeks and found out nobody welcomed them in. One older couple did, and thus Zeus and Hermes let them make one wish. Their wish was to die together, so Zeus and Hermes turned them into two oak trees. They could now live together for a long time.

Susan leaves for a nursing home, and Fred stays with a caretaker. When he is told that his children will pick him up, he does not want to go. ("Who will be here when Susan comes back?") It seems that the children remain at an impasse and are unable to resolve it with the best of intentions. Bob decides in a flash to get Fred a new cinnamon-colored cat ("Ginger"), faking that he has found her behind a tree. (In reality, "Ginger" has long been dead, but Fred has been asking for her.) Fred is elated that "Ginger" has been found, and this scene suddenly indicates a far more profound dementia than what had seemed apparent. The cat escapes, and the film ends abruptly, and in the end we do not know whether Fred moves out. When the credits came on, I thought to myself, maybe we should all turn into oak trees when the time comes.

A Final Word

Difficult behaviors in dementia are common. Delay in placement with good care could save billions of dollars annually, and efforts to keep patients at home do improve their quality of life. These two remarkable films show how children cope with their debilitated parents—debilitated from a dementing illness, left on their own with nowhere to go. But these are also parents unwilling to accept help, unable to cope, and spiraling into rapid self-neglect. These are the major themes, and these issues are where the strength of these films lies.

Further Reading

Caron CD, Ducharme F, Griffith J. Deciding on institutionalization for a relative with dementia: The most difficult decision for caregivers. *Can J Aging* 2006;25:193–205.

Klug MG, Volkov B, Muus K, Halaas GW. Deciding when to put grandma in the nursing home: Measuring inclinations to place persons with dementia. *Am J Alzheimers Dis Other Demen* 2012;27:223–27.

Smith GE, O'Brien PC, Ivnik RJ, Kokmen E, Tangalos EG. Prospective analysis of risk factors for nursing home placement of dementia patients. *Neurology* 2001;57:1467–73.

Yaffe K, Fox P, Newcomer R, et al. Patient and caregiver characteristics and nursing home placement in patients with dementia. *JAMA* 2002;287:2090–97.

EXPERIMENTATION IN FILM

Extreme Measures (1996); starring Hugh Grant, Gene Hackman, Sarah Jessica Parker, and David Morse; directed by Michael Apted, written by Tony Gilroy; distributed by Columbia Pictures.

Rating

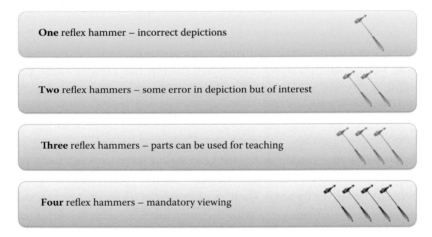

One reflex hammer – incorrect depictions

Two reflex hammers – some error in depiction but of interest

Three reflex hammers – parts can be used for teaching

Four reflex hammers – mandatory viewing

Criticism and Context

Mad scientists and physicians—recognized by a wide-eyed and flyaway-hairdo appearance—have been known since the era of silent film. Later, when scientists spoke in the movies, they often had a German accent, which brings to mind Dr. Strangelove (played by Peter Sellers) in Stanley Kubrick's masterpiece. Mad physicians are mostly found in horror films, most of which have to do with creating humanoid monsters. Both Dr. Frankenstein (from Mary Shelley's book *Frankenstein)* and Dr. Moreau (from H.G. Wells's book, *The Island of Dr. Moreau*) have been personified in film and seen experimenting and surgically reshaping monstrous figures.

Extreme Measures is iconic because for the first time a film suggests there might be wildly experimenting neurologists out there. The film starts with Dr. Guy Luthan (played by Hugh Grant) noticing "strange symptoms" in a homeless patient admitted to the emergency department. It becomes rapidly clear that the neurologist, Lawrence Myrick (Gene Hackman), performs experiments on homeless patients in order to find a cure for spinal cord injury. The film addresses several unethical behaviors beyond the obvious lack of informed consent.

The film is quite up-front with its premise when Myrick tells Luthan that the homeless (with no benefit to society) can be "heroes" by providing possible cures to millions, even if it leads to their own deaths. This key conversation explains the title of the film. Myrick declares that he has no time to conduct trials for a promising new drug in rats or chimpanzees.

Quotable Lines of Dialogue

Extreme Measures	
Neurologist, Dr. Lawrence Myrick	*People die every day, and for what? For nothing. What do we do? What do you do? You take care of the ones you think you can save. Good doctors do the correct thing, but great doctors have the guts to do the right thing.*

Introducing new therapies to healthy human controls is unusual without the setting of a randomized controlled trial, and the scenario in *Extreme Measures* is not only highly improbable, but frankly criminal. Without giving away too much of the plot, this eventually leads to a major confrontation and after the neurologist is accidentally shot, the protagonist gets the full research data from his wife and he decides to enter a neurology residency. Here the film supports the premise that the therapy might work but for the fact that the wrong method was used. It just needs another try.

The film has everything that can go wrong in the professionalism and ethics of neurology research. *Extreme Measures* avoids the major principles of research (of course for dramatic purposes), which are do no harm, full disclosure, and the right to refuse participating in research without consequences for future care. In fact, it ignores all major ethical principles.

The American College of Physicians has summarized their principles of medical professionalism (Table 4.3). Financial conflicts of interest continue to be a major concern in medicine, and medical decisions may still

TABLE 4.3   Principles of Medical Professionalism

1.	Commitment to professional competence
2.	Commitment to honesty with patients
3.	Commitment to patient confidentiality
4.	Commitment to maintaining appropriate relations with patients
5.	Commitment to improving quality of care
6.	Commitment to improving access to care
7.	Commitment to a just distribution of finite resources
8.	Commitment to scientific knowledge
9.	Commitment to maintaining trust by managing conflicts of interest
10.	Commitment to professional responsibilities

Source: ABIM Foundation, Medical professionalism in the new millennium: A physician charter. *Ann Intern Med* 2002;136:243–46.

be influenced by monetary considerations. Patient self-determination or autonomy—although a major principle—has been taken to another level in this movie, but it is also suggested that data of unethical research can be used and analyzed.

Unfortunately, the history of medicine is blemished by unethical research, notably the Tuskegee syphilis experiments, which studied the natural history of untreated syphilis. The participants were not aware that they had syphilis, and they were not treated with penicillin. Similarly, multiple radiation experiments on unwitting subjects are on record, and these are summarized in the report "Three Decades of Radiation Experiments on U.S. Citizens." Most notorious are the Nazi human neurologic experiments that included head injury experiments in children, hypothermia experiments on captured Russian troops, and brain studies at high altitudes. Currently, clinical research is strongly regulated, and academic centers train clinical researchers through close mentorship. All research protocols are overseen by institutional review boards that demand close record keeping.

A Final Word

Respect for each individual person is a major moral principle guiding the ethics of research. This means that persons are never asked to be research subjects against their will or coerced into participation. Vulnerable populations must be protected by proxy (a surrogate decision maker). The concept of *informed consent* relies on several prerequisites: (a) the person has been given all information needed; (b) the person has a good understanding of the pros and cons; and (c) the person is not being deceived. Vulnerable populations include patients with Alzheimer's disease, critically ill patients, sedated and agitated patients, and of course any comatose patient. Participation in research should always be voluntary. Waivers are not allowed if the researcher does not have the time to reach the relatives of the person subjected to research, although waivers are allowed in emergency treatments that potentially could benefit the patient.

Further Reading

Bernat JL. Restoring medical professionalism. *Neurology* 2012;79:820–27.

Frayling C. *Mad, Bad and Dangerous?: The Scientist and Cinema*. London: Reaktion Books, 2005.

Ringel SP, Steiner JF, Vickrey BG, Spencer SS. Training clinical researchers in neurology: We must do better. *Neurology* 2001;57:388–92.

Smithline HA, Gerstle ML. Waiver of informed consent: A survey of emergency medicine patients. *Am J Emerg Med* 1998;16:90–91.

COMPASSION FAILURE IN FILM

The Death of Mr. Lazarescu (2005); starring Ioan Fiscuteanu and Luminita Gheorghiu; written and directed by Cristi Puiu (cowritten by Razvan Radulescu); Un Certain Regard Award at Cannes Film Festival; distributed by Tartan USA.

Rating

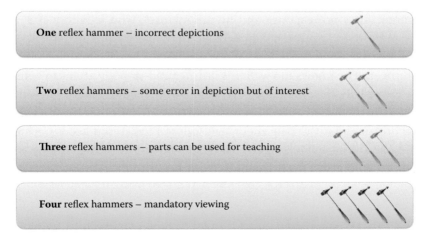

One reflex hammer – incorrect depictions

Two reflex hammers – some error in depiction but of interest

Three reflex hammers – parts can be used for teaching

Four reflex hammers – mandatory viewing

Criticism and Context

Ideally, physicians care for their patients' well-being and do not discriminate; they treat everyone the same and contribute to healing of the patient. That is true in most circumstances and in most hospitals. However, such a constant commitment is difficult and must be taught. Burnout of physicians may occur with overwhelmingly high workload, lack of restorative rest, and considerable emotional burden. There is one major film that addresses all of these problems, and without hesitation is recommended as required viewing for all neurologists, neurosurgeons, and perhaps even all physicians. The film shows a lack of humanity in a hospital system where the staff has been overcome by gruff and sarcastic behavior. Based on a true story when an ambulance in Romania that tried to admit a patient to various hospitals, all of which refused to admit him, the patient was ultimately left to die on the street.

The Death of Mr. Lazarescu is many layers deep. Several themes are threaded throughout the story, but in the end the viewer is confronted by the lack of appropriate neurologic and neurosurgical care. Dante Remus Lazarescu (played by the renowned theater actor Ioan Fiscuteanu) is a widowed retired engineer in his senior years. His daughter has left for the United States, and he lives with his cats. His pension is handled by his sister, who takes most of it. He has been a heavy drinker, predominantly of mastropol (homemade alcohol). He lives in a run-down apartment in Bucharest, Romania, and the film opens with him calling for an ambulance because of headache and vomiting. Nobody seems to be alarmed, and no ambulance shows up late on this Saturday night. He goes to a neighbor (after no response and no ambulance), who tells him it is his ulcer. When Mr. Lazarescu vomits blood in the neighbor's apartment, the neighbor tells him it is Mallory–Weiss syndrome. Yes, Lazarescu has been drinking, but he knows too well this is different—nobody seems to believe him. Eventually the ambulance arrives, and the medic Mioara (played by the equally renowned actor Luminita Gheorghiu), becomes his "guardian angel" throughout the long night that follows. Lazarescu keeps on mentioning headache, but it is again all attributed to his drinking. Mioara tries to find an emergency department that can help him.

Upon arrival at the first hospital, the emergency physician tells him again, when he complains of a headache, that he should stop drinking. The emergency physician gets irritated, pokes in his right upper quadrant, notices an enlarged liver, and concludes that there is little he can do. Lazarescu is told to go elsewhere when an acute multitrauma comes in.

In another hospital, an astute young physician detects a subtle arm drift and calls for a neurologist, who calls for an emergent CT, but he is told he still has to wait for 3 hours. (The neurologist examination is remarkable, and it is described in detail in Chapter 2.) Gradually, Lazarescu becomes more and more sleepy. The neurosurgeon arrives after the CT scan shows a subdural hematoma and a presumably cancerous mass in the liver. At this point, the film picks up speed and becomes far more dramatic in showing appalling physician behavior. The neurosurgeon seems uninterested in proceeding but asks him to sign a consent form. ("If I operate without his signature, I go to jail.") A conflict arises between the neurosurgeon and the medic when she suggests the need for a rapid operation. He tells her to go to a different hospital. (He also sarcastically suggests driving around for an hour, because when the patient becomes comatose, a doctor does not need a signature.) Finally, in the last hospital, the need for surgery is recognized, and we see him naked on a stretcher getting washed and head shaved. By now, he is deeply stuporous. The title of the film implies he dies, but we do not see it.

There is little compassionate care for Mr. Lazarescu. (His first name, Dante, is allegorical, and his family name sounds very much like the biblical person Lazarus.) Lazarescu's dignity and autonomy are neglected—all because he is an alcoholic and smelly. He is an extremely vulnerable patient in an overstretched medical system where egotism is rampant. The informed consent is the worst of its kind. There is an attempt to help him sign while someone supports his hand and even attempts to do it for him before he throws out the sheets of paper. He is also told that the surgery is nothing more than surgery for an appendectomy. The medic, who follows him through all the niches of all the hospitals, seems the last hope in this Orwellian-Kafkaesque world.

Quotable Lines of Dialogue

The Death of Mr. Lazarescu	
Neurosurgeon	*You are not in a coma. You are not lethargic. You feel a bit sleepy. Me too. It is 3:05 a.m.*
Emergency physician	*Hospitals are full of people like you that soak their brains in alcohol and batter their wives and kids.*
Lazarescu	*My head hurts, Doctor.*
Emergency physician	*Good, that means you have one.*

What can we learn from this remarkable film? Poor working conditions—such as those depicted in the film—will lead to dissatisfaction and dwindling of compassion, often first recognized by sarcasm. This impact on the quality of care may result in quick, poorly thought-out decisions (i.e., all alcoholics with headache are hung over) and conflicts with coworkers (i.e., "How do you dare to question me?"), and *The Death of Mr. Lazarescu* demonstrates that phenomenally.

The *Oxford English Dictionary* defines the term *compassion fatigue* as "apathy or indifference towards the suffering of others or to charitable causes acting on their behalf, typically attributed to seemingly frequent appeals for assistance, esp. donations; hence a diminishing public response to frequent appeals." It involves all healthcare workers, including clergy, and failure to remedy an unworkable situation (such as Ceausescu's damaged Romania) only perpetuates this miserable situation.

The director's intention was to depict the fear of dying alone. The film shows the worst of medicine. Dante Lazarescu is funneled through a hellish medical system devoid of compassion and inadequate in its resources. With every passing hour, Lazarescu gradually deteriorates from a subdural hematoma and develops hemiparesis and dysarthria, and finally to aphasia and drowsiness—all not recognized by caregivers. The medic's persistence finally results in finding a hospital, but by then it is too late.

A Final Word

The message of the film is that overburdened healthcare workers may overlook major health issues, especially when the person needing care is outside the boundaries of what is expected as normal care. In this case, the reluctance to deal with an unkempt, vomiting patient—instead handing the patient off to another facility—proved to be a fatal mistake. Most hospitals in Romania are not this way; most hospitals in many other countries are not this way; but this scenario definitely could occur anywhere. Does this self-important physician behavior have a familiar ring? I am afraid that, sometimes, it does.

This film should be required viewing for all neurologists and neurosurgeons. It is my personal favorite; see Chapter 7. This moral tale also tells us everything about the need for education in bedside manners. For many decades there has been a concern about the loss (or erosion) of the art of medicine, and while that might be partly true, medical schools recognize that their students need to understand that the onset of disease is usually unexpected. The other end of this equation is a deeply suffering human being (and family) confronted with an urgent need to deal with the disease. I always cringe when I hear a resident tell me he has a "great case" to present.

Further Reading

Crowan RM, Trzeciak S. Clinical review: Emergency department overcrowding and the potential impact on the critically ill. *Crit Care* 2005;9:291–95.

Epp K. Burnout in critical care nurses: A literature review. *Dynamics* 2012;23:25–31.

Huber C. A tale from the Bucharest hospitals. *Cinema Scope* 2006:6.

Hyman SA, Michaels DR, Berry JM. Risk of burnout in perioperative clinicians. *Anesthesiology* 2011;114:1–2.

Page DW. Are surgeons capable of introspection? *Surg Clin North Am* 2011;91:293–304, vii.

Riding A. "Death of Mr. Lazarescu" comes after a bout of hypochondria. *The New York Times.* April 23, 2006.

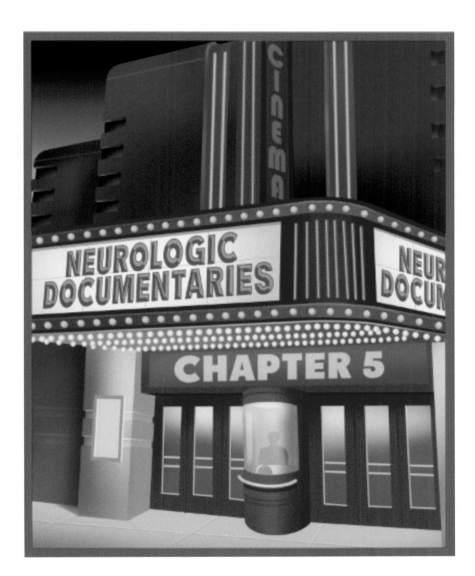

CHAPTER 5

Neurologic Disorders in Documentary Film

It kind of grounds you, it brings you back to reality.

*But You Still Look so Well: More Living
With Multiple Sclerosis* (2012)

INTRODUCTION OF MAIN THEMES

Fiction film gives a dramatized portrayal of neurologic disease, while documentary film portrays reality. Some fiction films—particularly those that belong to the art-house category—mimic reality very well (e.g., *Amour* [2012]), but it could be said that neurology is best represented in documentary form. But is it? It is well recognized by film scholars that documentaries may paradoxically have a much higher "deception factor." Because viewers accept material shown in documentaries as reality, they may not recognize that the reality behind these documentaries may be far more complicated than what is shown. Documentary filmmakers may have an agenda, and they may make their film to pose some difficult questions or to show us a difficult situation, but this is mostly for shock value. There also may be reenacted scenes that give the illusion of reality. For good reason, then, this kind of creative work may be viewed with some healthy suspicion. It may be what film critic Geoffrey O'Brien called "movies with documents."

There are several recent notable medical documentaries, and they may involve healthcare systems (*Sicko* [2007]) or lack thereof (*The Waiting Room* [2012], *The English Surgeon* [2007]), the food we eat and the food that makes us sick (*Food, Inc.* [2008]), and attacks on the pharmaceutical industry (*Big Buck, Big Pharma* [2006]). Some have admirably addressed the loneliness of dying of cancer (*Dying at Grace* [2003]) and AIDS (*How to Survive a Plague* [2012]). Each of these documentaries has unearthed potential problems in the practice of medicine or prevention of disease. However, documentaries may not necessarily influence public opinion, create awareness, or have the audience see the topic from a new angle.

There are multiple short documentaries on neurologic disease, usually made by patient organizations. Some neurologic documentaries are shown in disability film festivals—most notably, the New York disability film festival (www.reelabilities.org). This festival primarily features films by and about people with disabilities and exists to "explore, discuss and celebrate the diversity of our shared human experience." In many films the difference between developmental intellectual disability and autism is not sufficiently clear.

Some serious full-length neurologic documentaries have emerged. This is a consequence of more readily available footage as a result of user-friendly cameras. Documentaries may be problematic if they involve filming of persons who are not aware of their disease—a topic for consideration in the ethics of documentary filmmaking. Documentaries of patients with severe cognitive impairment create an immediate ethical concern. How do we know that the patient would be agreeable to be filmed even if the family agrees? However, nothing of this sort is apparent in the selection presented in this chapter, and documentary filmmakers are, for the most part, careful about these ethical concerns. Matters are usually presented in a more serious vein, and filmmakers do not make light of people's disabilities.

Neurologic documentaries may involve partly eradicated disease, with poliomyelitis as a great example. The mystery of lytico-bodig disease on the island of Guam in the 1950s with its features of amyotrophic lateral sclerosis, Parkinson disease, and dementia (and ceasing to exit) is recently featured in *The Illness and Odyssey* (2013).

Sentimentalization of neurologic illness is also a potential concern. Some documentaries show the full devastation of a life-threatening neurologic disease. These may be very difficult to watch, and some viewers may want to look away, or wonder why we even would want to see these films.

In this chapter, full-length documentaries on major brain injury and progressive neurologic disease are explored. Major topics include dementia, amyotrophic lateral sclerosis, multiple sclerosis, stroke, and rehabilitation of traumatic brain injury. I also discuss filmmakers with neurologic disease, filmmakers with parents with neurologic disease, and filming in nursing homes or in a patient's home environment.

The selection of documentaries presented here is not necessarily complete, because many neurologic disorders are not filmed in a documentary format, but each contains useful teaching material and are recommended viewing for all neurologists and healthcare workers involved in neurorehabilitation.

DEMENTIA IN DOCUMENTARY FILM

You're Looking at Me Like I Live Here and I Don't (2012); written and directed by Scott Kirschenbaum; distributed by You're Looking at Me LLC.

Rating

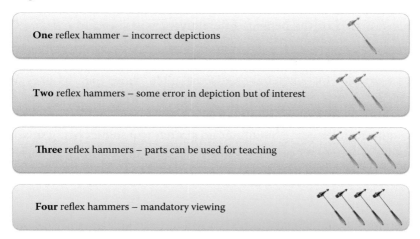

One reflex hammer – incorrect depictions

Two reflex hammers – some error in depiction but of interest

Three reflex hammers – parts can be used for teaching

Four reflex hammers – mandatory viewing

The Genius of Marian (2013); directed by Banker White; distributed by Capital Film Fund.

Rating

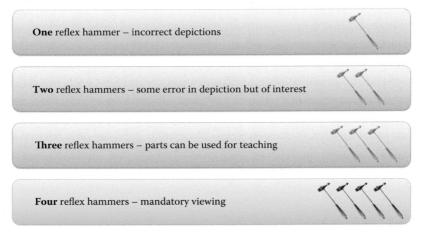

One reflex hammer – incorrect depictions

Two reflex hammers – some error in depiction but of interest

Three reflex hammers – parts can be used for teaching

Four reflex hammers – mandatory viewing

Criticism and Context

Alzheimer's disease is widespread, and thus we can hope for a penetrating film that shows its clinical course and its consequences. Most documentary films concentrate on caregivers facing the burden of managing the behavioral problems of patients still living at home with Alzheimer's disease. Usually the perspective is from the viewpoint of the caretaker, and the caretaker is often the narrator. Some TV documentaries have involved artists or the benefits of creative arts, as seen in *I Remember When I Paint* (2009). The filmmaker may choose, for dramatic purposes, the loss of creativity and thus the loss of what could have been. Documentaries on Alzheimer's disease often show that spouses and significant others end up caring for a person who has lost all of the personality traits that created their bond. It has been called ambiguous loss—physically missing but not dead, similar to a soldier being missing in action. These films can also show the reality of nursing homes, with all their benefits and drawbacks.

The documentary *You're Looking at Me Like I Live Here and I Don't* takes a different approach. This work was filmed inside the Traditions Alzheimer's Unit in Danville, California, and focuses on one nursing home resident, Lee Gorewitz, who is in her 70s (Figure 5.1a). The documentary opens with photos of Lee before her diagnosis, but no backstory is given. The filmmaker then simply shows her going from one activity to another. She is different from the other, more sedate residents. Acting as a tour guide of the nursing home, she hops around from place to place, talking spontaneously. She seems very comfortable, nonagitated, nonsedated, but she has no insight. Somewhat ironically, early in the documentary, the filmmaker asks her if she knows what Alzheimer's disease is. Her answer is complete gibberish. When she tries to read her nametag, she can only read her last name, but is able to spell it aloud.

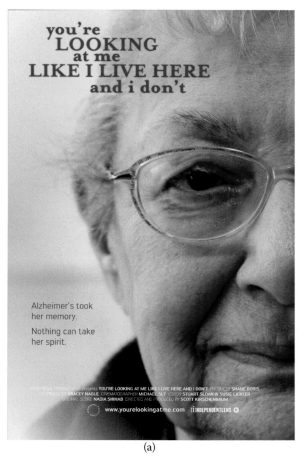

(a)

FIGURE 5.1   (a) Film poster of *You're Looking at Me Like I Live Here and I Don't*.

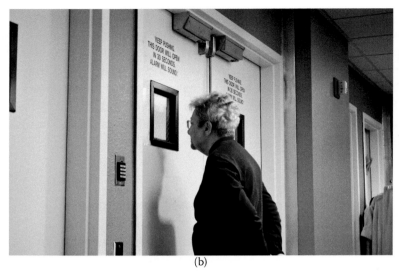
(b)

FIGURE 5.1 (*Continued*)   (b) Lee Gorewitz (before the exit door). (Used with permission from Scott Kirschenbaum.)

Quotable Lines of Dialogue

You're Looking at Me Like I Live Here and I Don't

Filmmaker	*What is Alzheimer's disease?*
Lee Gorewitz	*Alzheimer is the family of...uh...God, I have lost it. Alzheimer is the person that goes down and helps to help the person who does and gets to feel what is it once again. Alzheimer? That is kinda funny for me... weird...I guess I do not understand how you can have two together.*

Walking through the nursing home, Lee is pleasant, spry, and chuckling. When she meets one of the caregivers or nursing assistants, she asks, "Are you doing a simple thing that you do not have to do anymore?" When the caregiver responds, "What do you need?" Lee answers, "It all depends on how it goes along." She solo dances, snapping her fingers like a lounge singer, in front of the camera with music playing Frank Sinatra's *Somewhere Beyond the Sea*. The other residents are in varied stages of dementia, some participating in activities, some barely engaging, some just hunched over. When Lee comes across an older woman slumped over in a chair, she comments, "That one looks like it's dead."

A poignant moment comes when she looks at family photos and comments, seemingly lucid, "Here it is my family who are really doing nothing to help me (chuckles)…you always did it that way." When her deceased husband is mentioned, she comments, "How do I even say it? The air—was very good."

Her language deficit can be understood as speech devoid of specific content words (nouns and verbs), using only pronouns (his, it, they), and often she does not know what she is referring to. Speech is also convoluted, meandering, disjointed, and circumlocuting. This emptying out of speech and vocabulary is fairly characteristic in dementia, with patients answering in short sentences and showing nothing of the verbal sophistication known before to family members. Lee loses her train of thought frequently. Her language is best characterized as an aphasic dementia and not a primary progressive aphasia. She is not aware of her speech deficit.

The filmmaker shows how touching and happy some patients can be in a protected, closed environment. Lee tries to work the code of the exit door (Figure 5.1b) but is not frustrated when it does not work after she randomly punches in numbers. This remarkable minimalistic documentary shows that dementia may not always lead to a distressing situation, and a happier disposition may exist (at least for some time). Lee Gorewitz passed away in 2012.

The Genius of Marian is a documentary directed by Banker White, who films his mother Pam White (Figure 5.2) in the early stages of Alzheimer's disease. The title, *The Genius of Marian*, refers to a book Pam was writing about her mother (Marian), who was a painter. Marian developed Alzheimer's disease and stopped painting. Most of Marian's watercolor paintings are prominently present in this documentary. Pam was a year into the project, but at age 61 was also diagnosed with Alzheimer's disease. The film shows the considerable burden of care for Pam's husband, and thus does provide some new insights into these stages of Alzheimer's disease. It clearly shows the viewer that the early stages of Alzheimer's can be hard to define, and that advancement to other stages may become quickly apparent as months go by. Not much context is given to the viewer; however, the film does introduce the viewer to the gradual onset of deficits. In Pam's case, one of the most "shocking developments" for her family was that she could not figure out the tip on a restaurant check. Her son, a physician, adds that when he visited his parents, more deficits were gradually noted and that Pam behaved out of character, verbally attacking her husband. He prescribed her medication to be "calm and happy." The documentary shows her life fading out, more frequent awakening by her husband, and him trying to get her out of bed to dress her. Pam's husband is

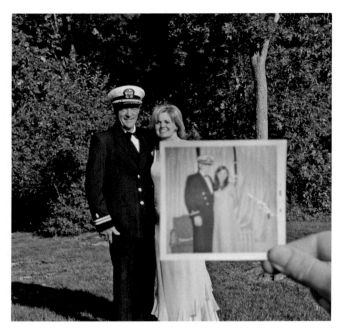

FIGURE 5.2   Pam White and her husband (and the years gone by). (Used with permission from Banker White.)

constantly by her side. ("I like to be with her. I don't mind doing it.") Most touching is Pam's remark that "I was quite distressed and upset about it, but it does not really matter. It does not really change anything, and I don't feel sad and I don't feel regret...." This disconnect and lack of insight is well represented. The documentary is notable because it shows a family trying to cope with the not-so-subtle dementia of a wife and mother. The disintegration of her mind is contrasted with beautiful, colorful, and warm watercolors, and these paintings provide some solace from what we are seeing so clearly here—early Alzheimer's disease in a genetically affected family.

Several other documentaries deserve mention. *The Forgetting: A Portrait of Alzheimer's* (2010) ⚞ is an Emmy Award-winning documentary showing the disease in its different stages, gradually progressing to its nadir. The film provides some useful medical background and shows the 1906 discovery of the disease by Alois Alzheimer—as head of his neuroanatomical laboratory—and his observation of "peculiar changes of the neurofibrils" in his key patient Auguste D. The documentary is narrated by family members, researchers, and clinicians. This film is somewhat difficult to watch, showing belligerent behavior as part of the relentless decline, until nothing more than an immobile, dazed body remains.

A similar approach is seen in *Extreme Love: Dementia* (2012) ⟪, where we visit Beatitudes, a special unit for dementia in a housing complex for seniors. It is part of the *BBC Extreme Love* series directed by Louis Theroux, a British journalist with a resumé of shocking documentaries. It shows some interesting aspects of care, such as "going along with an hallucination" and not telling a patient they will be a permanent resident, in order to avoid major upset. This documentary suggests that the husband of one of the couples considers divorcing his wife to have the state pay her medical bills.

Other recent documentaries on dementia are *Vergiss mein Nicht* (2012) and *Mam* (2009). A major recent project is the series *Living with Alzheimer's* (LivingwithAlz.org), which includes several short documentaries.

Two recent documentaries explore music and Alzheimer's disease. Alive Inside (2014) ⟪⟪ is about Dan Cohen, a social worker, who surreptitiously found that some patients with Alzheimer's disease in nursing homes responded extraordinarily to their favorite music, using an iPod. The emotional link to music is very convincing when you see two of the characters becoming markedly animated with music. Alive Inside is a deeply moving documentary about doing well with surprisingly little resources. Music may be soothing and therapeutic for many patients who otherwise would need psychotropic medication. Glenn Campbell...I'll Be Me (2014) ⟪⟪ is about Campbell's farewell tour after being diagnosed with Alzheimer's disease. The striking feature is the contrast between his inability to function in normal life situations and his glorious presence on stage—at least to a certain point, where it all falls apart.

A Final Word

We are in the midst of a steep increase in elderly patients with dementia, with healthcare costs three times more than for patients without dementia. There is no cure or even a solid understanding of Alzheimer disease. Research has focused on a beta-amyloid problem (the "Baptists") and a tau problem (the "Tauists"). Others maintain there is an environmental (toxic) cause. Millions of Americans provide unpaid care for their loved ones, and many have stopped working or reduced their working hours as a result. These documentaries elucidate the toll this takes. They also show the nursing home and administrative nursing staff and their quality in meeting the needs of patients.

Further Reading

Bullock R. The needs of the caregiver in the long-term treatment of Alzheimer disease. *Alzheimer Dis Assoc Disord* 2004;18 Suppl 1:S17–23.

Chivers S. *The Silvering Screen: Old Age and Disability in Cinema.* Toronto: University of Toronto Press, 2011.

Confronting the crisis in dementia care. *Lancet Neurol* 2009;8:413.

Hill E. Coping with ambiguous loss. *The Lancet Neurology* 2012;11:215.

Kukull WA. The growing global burden of dementia. *The Lancet Neurology* 2006;5:199–200.

Mudher A, Lovestone S. Alzheimer's disease: do tauists and baptists finally shake hands? *Trends Neurosci* 2002;25:22–26.

Swinnen A. Dementia in documentary film: mum by Adelheid Roosen. *Gerontologist* 2013;53:113–122.

Wijdicks EFM. Gimme shelter and an iPod. *Lancet Neurol* 2014, In press.

Wijdicks EFM. Not gentle on his mind. *Lancet Neurol* 2014, In press.

HUNTINGTON DISEASE IN DOCUMENTARY FILM

Do You Really Want to Know? (2012); written and directed by John Zaritsky; distributed by Optic Nerve Films.

Rating

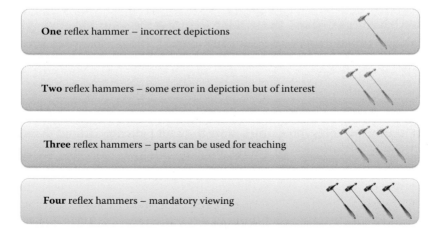

One reflex hammer – incorrect depictions

Two reflex hammers – some error in depiction but of interest

Three reflex hammers – parts can be used for teaching

Four reflex hammers – mandatory viewing

Criticism and Context

Neurogenetics has found its way into the movies (Chapter 3), but rarely into documentary film. Most familial neurodegenerative diseases have no cure, and there is no medication that can notably slow down or delay the manifestations of the disorder. It would seem that for filmmakers, there may not be much to show other than the relentless decline of the patient. However, further characterization of the genetic code of these disorders, and eventually prediction of its later appearance through laboratory testing, has become a reality.

Some scientists have stated that precision (individualized) medicine is just around the corner, and if so, this could create immediate ethical problems with neurologic disorders of late onset. Accurate prediction (knowing if you will get it) varies for each of the neurologic disorders, and actual testing may involve insufficiently validated biomarkers.

One disease in this category is Huntington's disease, and the filmmaker has found a way to address the major problems with these decisions in the documentary *Do You Really Want to Know?* (Figure 5.3). Since the gene was discovered in 1993, genetic testing has become available. Genetic testing for Huntington's disease now is able to prediagnose some family members with a high probability, although nothing can be done to prevent the onset of the disease. Genetic testing has outrun understanding of the pathogenesis and treatment of the disease. Huntington's disease is a prime example of this medical quandary.

Huntington's disease is caused by the expansion of a trinucleotide (cyto-sine-adenine-guanine [CAG]) sequence on chromosome 4. This expansion within the Huntington gene results in an abnormally damaging protein. It is known that even if a patient tests positive, it cannot be predicted with 100% certainty that the disease will develop, because some patients with certain CAG length may be spared.

Huntington's disease is a neurodegenerative disease that progresses over many years and includes the development of myoclonus, chorea, dys-tonia, and rigidity as well as irritability and psychosis. Eventually, it may also lead to obsessive-compulsive behavior and depression. Hypomania is well recognized in patients with Huntington's disease. There are a num-ber of medications that are successful in muting the responses of many of these symptoms.

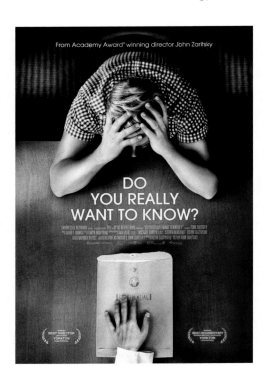

FIGURE 5.3   Film poster of *Do You Really Want to Know?* (Used with permission from Kevin Eastwood, producer.)

The motor symptoms of chorea (when awake) are constantly present and may involve head movements and tongue protrusion. There is often difficulty starting a movement, and dystonia may occur (abnormal positioning and tics). Walking is unsteady with ataxia features, and may also include dystonic posturing. Psychiatric symptoms include a combination of irritability and apathy followed by cognitive decline. Hypersexuality is common. The last clinical stage is marked by devastating motor symptoms, full dependence on others for care, and marked dementia. Nursing home placement is typical.

Do You Really Want to Know? is the first comprehensive documentary that addresses the symptoms of Huntington's disease and its penetration into families. The documentary goes through the difficult decisions that three different families have to make. The three key persons who are followed throughout the film are John Roder, Jeff Carroll, and Theresa Monahan.

John calls it a "genetic sentence." John is a scientist and has periods of severe chorea. He knew it ran in his family, but he and his wife decided to have two children, hoping that they would not pass on the gene. In 1993, when he was asymptomatic, he got tested, expecting a negative result, but the result was positive. In this documentary, it is 10 years since his diagnosis and he is impaired by chorea, dystonia, and spasticity.

A second key person in the documentary is Jeff Carroll, who decides to have the test, and he tests positive. When his wife becomes pregnant (both times), they decide to test prenatally, and fortunately both children are negative. Jeff became a researcher in Dr. Michael Hayden's laboratory, an internationally known Huntington's research facility in Canada.

Quotable Lines of Dialogue

Do You Really Want To Know?

Jeff   *You're never going to not know your status again. You can never turn back the clock and go to "maybe" again. You are always going to know one way or the other for sure.*

The third person is Theresa Monahan, a woman with a strong family history of Huntington's disease, who decides not to get tested despite her husband urging her to do so. However, at some point she proceeds with testing without informing her husband. He is kept in the dark for months while she knows that the test results are negative for Huntington's disease, effectively clearing her. For her, despite testing negative, this situation caused a stressful period, during which she waited for months to tell her husband (she felt she deceived him by not telling him she was getting tested).

The documentary provides important statistical data and a good overview of what Huntington's disease entails. Huntington's chorea, or Huntington's disease, is an autosomal-dominant disease. The prevalence of Huntington's disease has remained about 4–10/100,000. The disorder usually presents between the ages of 30 and 50, but most family members are aware of the disorder as a result of its considerable penetrance, with half the children of an affected family testing positive. Theresa's family is shown and provides a good example. Her grandfather was one of ten children, five of whom died from Huntington's disease, and her mother was one of seven children, four of whom died from Huntington's disease. Theresa calls herself "lucky."

It is known that only 5% to 10% of individuals at risk test themselves for Huntington's disease, even though predictive testing has been available for at least two decades. In general, females choose testing more than males, and the explanation is probably related to their reproductive decision-making process. However, surprisingly, the decision of whether to have offspring does not seem to be much different from those who carry the gene than for those who do not.

The film suggests the risk of suicide, but in general there has been a decrease in suicides in patients who have tested positive. This is relevant because depression is common in this population and often requires treatment (psychopharmacy and psychological help). The risk of suicide is highest around the testing period. Depression may even be in the preclinical stage when the uncertainty is the greatest. A related diagnostic problem is that Huntington's disease may present with psychiatric symptomatology before hyperkinesia or chorea starts.

A Final Word

Testing is available, but young individuals (<18 years) or those with severe psychiatric illnesses are excluded. In practice, very few proceed with testing for the disease. Most family members need a multidisciplinary approach before testing (geneticist, psychologist/psychiatrist, and neurologist), and this usually is set up in specialty clinics. The mean duration of Huntington's disease is about 15 years, and thus close care is needed.

This remarkable film about a rare neurologic disease admirably shows the major aspects of the disease and the dilemmas families face. Many decisions—wanting to know, not wanting to know, or wanting to know and not telling anyone—is how vulnerable humans respond to these tremendous uncertainties.

It remains unclear if there is any benefit in testing for Huntington's disease, but now that a test is available, family members have the right to know. Individuals may improve their well-being, and there is lower prevalence of depression in the group that decided to go ahead with genetic testing. When genetic testing becomes more commonplace, these decisions could apply to any late-onset neurodegenerative disease.

Further Reading

Almqvist EW, Bloch M, Brinkman R, Craufurd D, Hayden MR. A worldwide assessment of the frequency of suicide, suicide attempts, or psychiatric hospitalization after predictive testing for Huntington disease. *Am J Hum Genet* 1999;64:1293–1304.

Hans MB, Koeppen AH. Huntington's chorea: Its impact on the spouse. *J Nerv Ment Dis* 1980;168:209–14.

Hayden MR. Predictive testing for Huntington's disease: The calm after the storm. *Lancet* 2000;356:1944–45.

Kessler S, Bloch M. Social system responses to Huntington disease. *Fam Process* 1989;28:59–68.

Krukenberg RC, Koller DL, Weaver DD, Dickerson JN, Quaid KA. Two decades of Huntington disease testing: Patient's demographics and reproductive choices. *J Genet Couns* 2013;22:643–53.

Ross CA, Tabrizi SJ. Huntington's disease: From molecular pathogenesis to clinical treatment. *Lancet Neurol* 2011;10:83–98.

Tibben A. Predictive testing for Huntington's disease. *Brain Res Bull* 2007;72:165–71.

MULTIPLE SCLEROSIS IN DOCUMENTARY FILM

When I Walk (2013); directed by Jason DaSilva, written by Jason DaSilva and Alice Cook; distributed by Long Shot Factory.

Rating

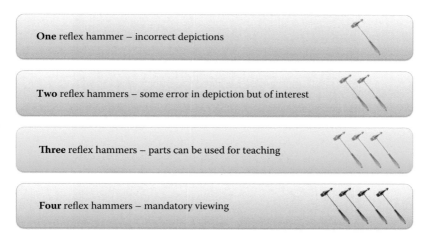

One reflex hammer – incorrect depictions

Two reflex hammers – some error in depiction but of interest

Three reflex hammers – parts can be used for teaching

Four reflex hammers – mandatory viewing

Criticism and Context

When I Walk is a diarist's documentary of 7 years' progression from primary progressive multiple sclerosis (MS) (Figure 5.4). Progressive MS is a universally progressive spinal disease. Clear criteria have been developed, and there is considerable interest in treatment of MS using therapies that include neuroprotection and myelin repair. The disease is rapidly progressive—time of onset to using a cane for walking is a median of 7 to 8 years. More recent studies report 14 years, with no clear explanation for the further delay.

The director of this film, Jason DaSilva, has several short films and feature-length documentary films to his credit. This personal documentary is a major accomplishment by a skilled filmmaker who lets us experience with

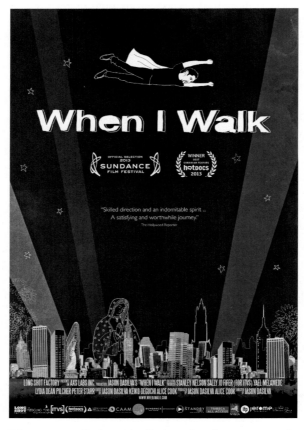

FIGURE 5.4   Film poster of *When I Walk*. (Used with permission from Long Shot Factory.)

him his progressive MS, the rapid changes over time, and all the major practical consequences of the disease for a young, vibrant person. Interwoven throughout the documentary is animation that calls attention to the burden of MS. DaSilva is diagnosed with MS, and we are first introduced to him when his legs give way during a vacation in the Caribbean. This occurs in the opening scene, when he is watching planes land with a few friends (ironically he points to a sign that warns of injury when spotting plane landings).

The film shows the initial stages of primary progressive MS. A brief interlude shows how primary progressive MS is defined and how it is considered an immunological disorder. Coping with the diagnosis of MS is presented in a fairly straightforward, unsentimental way. His mother explains that it could be worse, and compares it—as many people do when newly diagnosed—with other, more severe, disorders. She tells him he could be in a worse place—"The places where people are stuck."

Next DaSilva is seen exercising in the gym, hoping that his case and progression will be different. But he soon is confronted with a reality. While he is seen having a Shriner's gait assessment of his spastic gait, he is already—to his surprise—introduced by one of the healthcare workers to the possibility of a wheelchair. He is shown brochures of wheelchair suppliers but wants little to do with it.

The documentary shows, step by step, the relentless progression of this type of MS. Soon we see DaSilva having difficulty on stairs, and he is in need of a cane for stability. His marked spastic ataxic walk is prominently shown (hence the title, *When I Walk*). This walking handicap prevents him from easily going out on weekend nights. In a moving moment, he tells the viewer that he has had his "share of beautiful women," but as his MS gets worse, the girls seem to have disappeared into thin air. (This is emphasized by showing pictures of faded-out faces of his prior girlfriends.) It speaks volumes for a person this young being so visibly disabled. His mother plays an important role, often bringing him back to reality, although she can at times be harsh. ("We are really alone in this world.")

Quotable Lines of Dialogue

When I Walk	
Jason	*I just start using a cane and they are already talking about wheelchairs.*
Mother	*Things are tough in life. Get real, you mollycoddled North American kid.*

The film shows DaSilva's rapid MS progression in a matter of years, with his walking at first assisted by a walker and then becoming impossible. His ability to walk understandably becomes a major obsession. He visits India, a place he had been years previously, but this time, with his walker, he notices that people are staring at him when he walks—a much different experience than when he visited before. For him, the biggest question is whether he is able to make the films that he was planning to make. He accepts that he won't be able to climb mountains (the documentary shows people climbing mountains) or even be able to run (the documentary shows people running with the bulls in Spain). Soon his vision becomes affected, and he develops difficulty focusing and has to stop a project while in India. This is the time that DaSilva tries alternative medicine that includes yoga, transmeditation, and ayurvedic medicine. Nothing changes.

DaSilva visits his grand-uncle who is 87 years old, and asks him if there is a family history of MS (there is none). His grandmother, a devout Catholic, suggests he go to Lourdes, which he does. After he bathes in the waters at Lourdes, he dreams of running. ("Maybe a century of my family prayers will get me out of this.") Nothing changes. The film also follows DaSilva in his search searching for controversial surgical procedures, and he proceeds with the opening of his apparently obstructed cerebral veins. Nothing changes.

He visits an MS support group, where he meets his future wife (and also co-writer of this documentary). Alice is much less affected by her MS and is able to assist him. The film shows them having fun riding a scooter around the Guggenheim Museum, going to Hawaii, and eventually marrying. Finally DaSilva's life changes.

The documentary argues for better access to public places and identifies the difficulty of finding accessible ramps. In one cartoon, a big, red, monstrous ramp is shown, and DaSilva drives the point across that he cannot hail a taxi, cannot take the subway, and is markedly restricted in his mobility despite a scooter. He eventually develops a website for accessible places and an app helping persons with a disability.

His relationship with Alice makes his "depressing" situation (in his mother's words) far more endurable, and they often ponder about living with the disease and making a life of their own, maintaining their desires and ambitions. Despite the progressive MS, difficulty getting pregnant, and miscarriage, the film ends on a positive note when Alice again becomes pregnant and an ultrasound shows a fully developed fetus.

This film gives a compelling and realistic view into this rare form of MS and grappling with its challenges and limitations. The majority of people with MS have a relapsing-remitting form. Although many will eventually go on to develop progressive MS—the primary progressive form is in 10%–20% of all patients with multiple sclerosis—it appears to be a different type not responsive to any type of therapy. Drug trials have generally been unsuccessful, possibly due to the rapid progression. The film emphasizes the lack of disease-modifying therapy, although successful symptomatic therapy is seldom mentioned. It brings to the fore the search for alternative medicines as well as interventions that are highly controversial and often plainly unsubstantiated, such as improvement of chronic impaired venous outflow of the central nervous system (which has been shown by the latest studies to be flawed).

This documentary is one of the first comprehensive films on MS, but there have been other documentaries on MS, notably *"But You Still Look So Well…" Living with Multiple Sclerosis* (2005 and its sequel in 2012), which emphasizes that many patients have no visible signs of disease, and their diagnosis does not seem to impact on their daily life in a major way. MS may not always visibly affect patients, and thus the topic may not lend itself to a full feature film unless the progression is dramatic. *A Certain Kind of Beauty* (2006) also involves a young patient with primary progressive MS.

A Final Word

When I Walk invites viewers into the experience of a young creative man with progressive MS. It focuses on one of the three main forms of progressive MS (primary progressive vs. relapsing-remitting and secondary progressive). Nothing can slow the progressive disability of the disease, but drugs are available to improve symptoms. The film shows some of the desperation and the desire to seek alternative or unproven therapies. The documentary is very effective in showing a progressive disease intertwined with the emotionality of having a supportive partner. It does exactly what a neurologic documentary should do—provide a valuable teaching resource.

Further Reading

Confavreux C, Vukusic S. Natural history of multiple sclerosis: A unifying concept. *Brain* 2006;129:606–16.

Khan O, Filippi M, Freedman MS, et al. Chronic cerebrospinal venous insufficiency and multiple sclerosis. *Ann Neurol* 2010;67:286–90.

Koch MW, Cutter G, Stys PK, Yong VW, Metz LM. Treatment trials in progressive MS: Current challenges and future directions. *Nat Rev Neurol* 2013;9:496–503.

Montalban X, Sastre-Garriga J, Filippi M, et al. Primary progressive multiple sclerosis diagnostic criteria: A reappraisal. *Mult Scler* 2009;15:1459–65.

Rice CM, Cottrell D, Wilkins A, Scolding NJ. Primary progressive multiple sclerosis: Progress and challenges. *J Neurol Neurosurg Psychiatry* 2013;84:1100–6.

Valdueza JM, Doepp F, Schreiber SJ, et al. What went wrong? The flawed concept of cerebrospinal venous insufficiency. *J Cereb Blood Flow Metab* 2013;33:657–68.

Wolinsky JS. The diagnosis of primary progressive multiple sclerosis. *J Neurol Sci* 2003;206:145–52.

MOTOR NEURON DISEASE IN DOCUMENTARY FILM

So Much So Fast (2006); directed by Steven Ascher and Jeanne Jordan; distributed by West City Films.

Rating

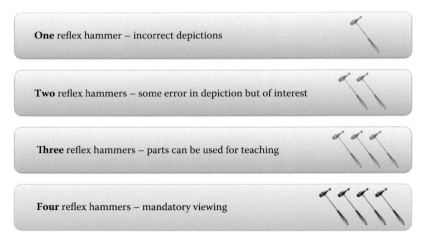

One reflex hammer – incorrect depictions

Two reflex hammers – some error in depiction but of interest

Three reflex hammers – parts can be used for teaching

Four reflex hammers – mandatory viewing

Living with Lew (2007); directed by Adam Bardach; distributed by Cinetic Media.

Rating

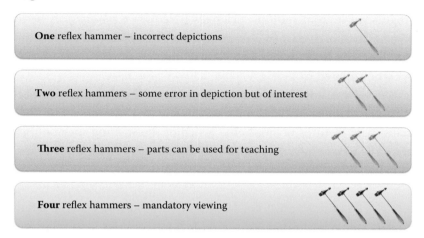

I Am Breathing (2013); directed by Emma Davie and Morag McKinnon; distributed by Scottish Documentary Institute.

Rating

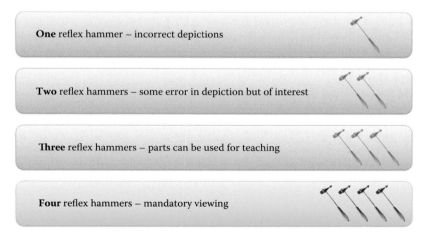

Criticism and Context

Amyotrophic lateral sclerosis (ALS) was first characterized by Charcot (Chapter 2). One of his patients with hysteria had major spasticity (upper motor neuron sign), which at autopsy was found to be caused by involvement of the lateral tracts of the spinal cord (*la sclérose latérale*), and he distinguished it from multiple sclerosis (*sclérose en plaques*). It became known as Charcot disease in Europe and the United Kingdom. Here in the United States, it is known as Lou Gehrig disease, for the famed baseball player who suffered from it.

ALS usually results in progressive wasting of the shoulder and pectoral muscles, atrophy in hand muscles (mostly first interossei and thenar muscles), and features of spasticity. Much of the wasting may be misinterpreted as weight loss, some of which occurs as a consequence of major swallowing difficulties.

Noninvasive ventilation will eventually fail to help the patient, typically when oropharyngeal weakness becomes prominent. Impaired glottis closure impairs maintenance of large lung volumes, and pharyngeal weakness may lead to occlusion of the upper airway. Oxygen desaturation despite maximal noninvasive settings is also an indicator that a tracheostomy is required. Many patients who choose a tracheostomy are young and have families, and some believe that holding on may allow a future treatment to cure the disorder. Tracheostomies are often performed emergently because no prior discussion has been entertained. This period of time is crucial for any ALS patient, and discussions are often postponed. If ventilation is not supported, most patients become unconscious or more unresponsive as a result of hypoxic-hypercarbic encephalopathy.

There are three major documentaries on ALS that needs attention and close examination. *So Much So Fast* follows the progression of ALS in Stephen Heywood. The film is also about the founding of the ALS Therapy Development Institute, which currently operates in Cambridge, Massachusetts, testing hundreds of drugs on genetically engineered mice. The film discusses in great detail a wish to accelerate drug trials, and it alleges "slow" progress in academia. The film starts with an important statement. "Back then [1993], there was only one rule: there was nothing you could do, no treatment, no surgery, no drugs."

Heywood was diagnosed with ALS at the age of 29. His brother, Jamy, started a foundation to find a treatment and became an aggressive negotiator. ("For a family, a diagnosis like that stops time; for Jamy, time sped up.") The film shows them discussing their ideas at the annual meeting of the Society of Neuroscience, and for Jamy, "It is a strange world. So many people obsessed with mice and rats." Jamy is determined to find ways to fight the establishment but also sees limitations. ("We are proposing ideas that can easily be shot down.")

The documentary shows two parallel stories—the difficulty of making progress in the laboratory and the relentless progression of Stephen's ALS. His wife tells us she can deal with a wheelchair, but him losing his voice is the hardest. He is finally seen on a ventilator, virtually locked in. He died in 2006 before the film's completion.

Living with Lew is about Lew, a movie director diagnosed with ALS. The documentary opens with a Lou Gehrig clip: "I might have been given a bad break, but I got an awful lot to live for." The film shows an upbeat Lew who cracks cynical jokes—for example, showing a nasal CPAP ("just like a fighter pilot") and the pills he is taking ("this is Haldol, LSD, peyote nugget, marijuana, etc."). In addition, he is taking multivitamins and tamoxifen ("at least I do not get breast cancer"). He is wearing a Lou Gehrig New York Yankees shirt.

The film shows interviews with healthcare workers in the Forbes Norris MDA/ALS Research Center, and there is a very succinct explanation of ALS and its programs. It mentions 3- to 5-year survival and 10% long-term survival (showing Stephen Hawking as an example). The film shows Lew in an advanced stage of ALS, but this documentary does not have the gravitas of the other documentaries. Some viewers may be put off by the dark sarcasm.

I Am Breathing is a documentary about Neil Platt, a 33-year-old architect with a familial form of ALS (father and grandfather). He is using a voice-recognition computer. The film pushes the boundaries of documentary filmmaking and follows him into the terminal stages and just before hospice care. His case is somewhat unique, with only 5% of all ALS cases being due to a familial form (ALS is a relatively frequent neurologic disease with 2/100,000). Platt died 14 months after the diagnosis (Figure 5.5).

The title *I Am Breathing* refers to the constant sound of the mechanical ventilator that is heard when the film opens. Platt is diagnosed at the age

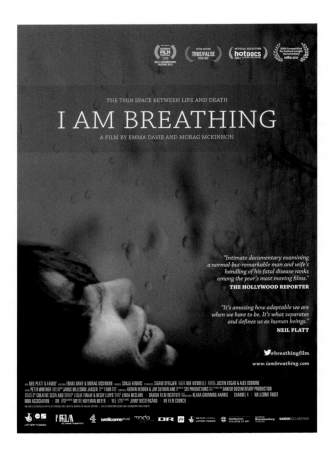

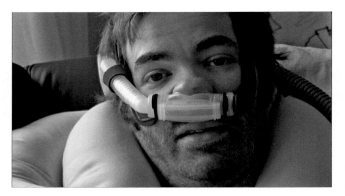

FIGURE 5.5 (a) Film poster of *I Am Breathing*; (b) Neil Platt on noninvasive mechanical ventilation. (Used with permission from Scottish Documentary Institute | SDI Productions Ltd.)

of 33, and we get to know him after several unusual remarks. He explains that he is looking into coffin catalogs and that he thinks of canceling his phone and shockingly tells the clerk that it's because he is dying. He challenges the viewer to try to fight an itch. This is all an introduction to what we are about to see—a young man struggling with a major illness while trying to keep up appearances and his sense of humor. Platt knows the cruel verdict all too well. The film shows him on CPAP and immobilized in a chair while being cared for by his young wife, Louise (her brave caring is extraordinary). Six months after his diagnosis, his hands stop working, and three months after that his legs stop working. His young child walks around in the room touching everything (including the power button of the ventilator).

His blog becomes his only outlet (http://plattitude.co.uk/), and he manages to dictate 100 blogs. The frustrating voice-recognition technology is notable here and becomes almost emblematic of the handicap he is facing. His blog is a long document that he has written for his son, Oscar, and he also ponders "the meaning of life and associated questions." ("I often ponder questions of such gravity and magnitude.") He is very clear that his advance directive is to not proceed with more intervention or surgical procedures when his voice disappears.

Quotable Lines of Dialogue

Neil Platt	*Just as the physical deterioration I have suffered is a result of motor neurone disease, so is the emotional deterioration of everyone touched by it. It pains me to think that the price being demanded by the disease is so high that not only does it reduce me to a talking head, but it eats away at the strong ties of family and friendship which ordinarily would withstand the most determined of attacks.*
Excerpt from Neil's Blog, *Plattitude*	

In an almost unbearable scene, Platt's airway obstructs and he has a choking episode, resulting in his wife using urgent percussion. Here his dysphagia becomes notable. This defining moment. This becomes inevitably the saddest part of the documentary. Platt is shown dictating his last words before he goes to hospice. "The reason I have chosen to go to the hospice tomorrow is to draw the curtain over what has been a devastating, degrading year and a half." He made the decision to remove the ventilator when he could not speak or swallow.

Neil Platt passed away on February 25, 2009. His son has a 50% chance of getting ALS. The film is a remarkable documentary on the rapid progression of young-onset ALS, and perhaps of any neurologic disease.

These three documentaries show different courses until the end. The outcome of ALS is an approximate 3-year survival in 50% of patients. The patient with onset in limbs seems to have less rapid progression than a patient starting the disease in the oropharyngeal region, and ALS starting in the legs has a slightly slower progression than upper early involvement of the arms. In Neil Platt's case, respiratory failure came relatively early, with largely preservation of speech and no severe dysphagia. (He is seen eating fish and chips while supported on nasal CPAP.) In Stephen Heywood's case, dysphagia came with dysarthria—as is more commonly seen. After gastrostomy placement, survival is still variable, usually about a year.

As is shown in these documentaries, ALS with early respiratory involvement does not necessarily imply a more progressive disease. Once respiration becomes involved in progressive ALS, the patient has a high likelihood of demise within a year unless mechanical ventilation is provided, as was the case for Stephen Heywood. (We see him in a final scene, mostly locked in with a tracheostomy and a respirator.)

Management of respiratory symptoms remains the most important determinant of outcome. A gastrostomy is often inserted if the patient is unable to maintain body weight or if there is frank dysphagia. Hypoxemia or hypercapnia is an important indication for noninvasive ventilation, and the majority of patients are able to tolerate noninvasive ventilation quite well. Noninvasive ventilation will improve both hypoxemia and hypercapnia, although it rarely normalizes these values.

ALS should be distinguished from primary lateral sclerosis (pyramidal signs only), progressive muscular atrophy (peripheral signs only), and progressive bulbar palsy (lower motor neuron involvement of speech and swallowing). Primary lateral sclerosis may have a median survival of 20 years, but the other disorders progress similarly to ALS. Outcome is also better in specialized clinics, largely due to much better symptom management. Weight loss also carries a poor prognosis, but even if gastrostomy placement leads to adequate feeding, it only improves quality of life.

A Final Word

This discussion has focused on three recent documentaries on ALS, each with a different perspective. Viewers are presented with the effects of a devastating neurologic illness that is almost unwatchable in the portrayal of its progression. Readers are best advised to turn to these documentaries, because fiction films (see Chapter 3) have made a clumsy mockery of the disease.

Further Reading

Ludolph AC, Brettschneider J, Weishaupt JH. Amyotrophic lateral sclerosis. *Curr Opin Neurol* 2012;25:530–35.

Platt N, Platt L. Plattitude. http://plattitude.co.uk/.

Rezania K, Roos RP. Spinal cord: Motor neuron diseases. *Neurol Clin* 2013;31:219–39.

Robberecht W, Philips T. The changing scene of amyotrophic lateral sclerosis. *Nat Rev Neurosci* 2013;14:248–64.

APHASIA AFTER STROKE IN DOCUMENTARY FILM

After Words (2013); directed by Vincent Straggas and cowritten by Jerome Kaplan; distributed by Flag Day Productions.

Rating

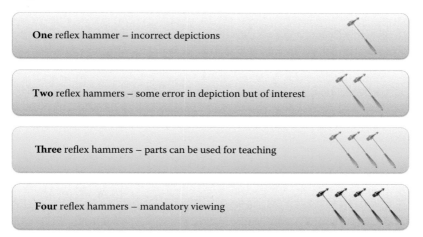

One reflex hammer – incorrect depictions

Two reflex hammers – some error in depiction but of interest

Three reflex hammers – parts can be used for teaching

Four reflex hammers – mandatory viewing

Picturing Aphasia (2006); directed by Mores McWreath; distributed by CreateSpace.

Rating

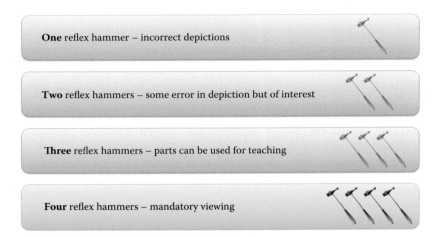

One reflex hammer – incorrect depictions

Two reflex hammers – some error in depiction but of interest

Three reflex hammers – parts can be used for teaching

Four reflex hammers – mandatory viewing

Aphasia (2010); starring Carl McIntyre; written and directed by Jim Gloster; distributed by Little Word Films.

Rating

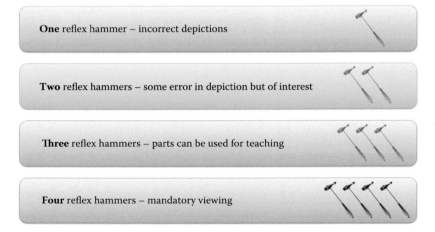

One reflex hammer – incorrect depictions

Two reflex hammers – some error in depiction but of interest

Three reflex hammers – parts can be used for teaching

Four reflex hammers – mandatory viewing

Criticism and Context

Documentaries about stroke typically involve coping with aphasia. There are no documentaries on the other disabilities that can accompany a stroke, such as the equally devastating loss of space orientation, neglect of the left side of the body, mood changes, and paralysis. Once a patient starts talking before the eye of the camera and the film demonstrates the impact of stroke on communication—something we take for granted—it invariably makes a strong impact on the viewing audience.

Aphasia can also be an almost invisible disability, especially those that are not accompanied by hemiplegia. This is often the case in posterior (fluent) aphasias, which may spare the motor cortex, and in patients with primary progressive aphasias. Our discussion here focuses on three recent major documentaries that address poststroke aphasia.

After Words includes the observations of several researchers who discuss the difficulties of family and close friends living with a person who is aphasic. The documentary is notable for its comprehensive explanation of aphasia. There is emphasis on therapy and recovery, and *After Words* is strong on how to improve quality of life in patients with aphasia.

After Words is a comprehensive look at aphasia caused mostly by stroke. It also briefly discusses primary progressive aphasia and presents one example of a patient with aphasia after a gunshot wound to the head. Several patients, spouses, and other family members are interviewed, and each patient clearly explains marked difficulties with language (Figure 5.6). All aspects

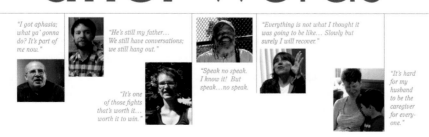

FIGURE 5.6   Patients with aphasia in scenes from *After Words*. (Kindly provided by Jerome Kaplan.)

of aphasia are discussed. Several neurologists are invited to comment and explain in simple ways what aphasia entails.

Various types of aphasia, not all of which are depicted in this film, present different severity levels. The additional challenge with receptive (or fluent) aphasia is that it often includes considerable deficits in comprehension, which complicate any effort to engage in meaningful dialogue. Dr. Marjorie Nicholas, Professor of Communication Sciences at the MGH Institute of Health Professions, provides an insightful description.

Quotable Lines of Dialogue

After Words

Marjorie Nicholas	*Imagine you are waking up in a foreign land, say Poland. They look around and everyone speaks Polish, and they do not understand the language; but they understand everything else about the world…and they cannot speak Polish.*

Speech-language pathologists are interviewed in this film, notably those in the team led by Jerome Kaplan, founder of the Aphasia Community Group. (Now in its 25th year, it is one of the oldest groups of its kind in the country.) They emphasize that patients with aphasia should be treated differently. Spouses (as well as other family members and caregivers) are faced with the task of figuring out what their loved one is attempting to communicate. Some patients mention that perseveration associated with severe expressive aphasia can be exhausting, and it shows.

The filmmaker Vincent Straggas recalls, "There is a struggle for them to communicate, and what one usually experiences is a more meaningful and thoughtful conversation. They are real and to the point, and don't waste time with idle chitchat."

After Words clearly dissects the abnormal components of aphasia and shows speech-language pathologists using a combination of music and speech therapy. (It is demonstrated that singing often improves speech and can be used as a tool.) This documentary takes a slightly different turn when an attorney states that one of her clients (a patient) was assaulted by an aide in a nursing home and then was found to be incompetent by a judge. This scene points out the risk of stigmatization in aphasic patients.

This documentary is a good resource for nonspecialists because it broadly explains and shows the challenges—and the sometimes devastating consequences—of aphasia.

Aphasia is acted and directed by Carl McIntyre. This documentary is narrated by Tim Parati and is used to support and promote his motivational speeches. Carl McIntyre was a theater actor who had a severe stroke, making it impossible for him to speak. The movie is also about errors in prognostication, when he is told that recovery would be within 6 months to a year, but little progress was made after 18 months. A combination of speech and occupational therapy has markedly improved his speech, and the documentary is largely about the will to overcome such a major disability.

The film—produced in association with the University of North Carolina at Chapel Hill and the Division of Speech and Hearing Sciences—has McIntyre reenact his stroke and its adverse effects. The lighthearted approach here feels awkward. The film shows him having difficulty getting words out and understanding written language—all in a comedic way. The film starts with him falling down on the floor, with his wife thinking he is "joking around." He then summarizes the time it takes to get treated, and "the stroke team had to be summoned from their secret hideout."

He "awakens" to find blurred faces over his bed, "as if I am in a Charlie Brown Halloween Special." The urgency of his stroke management is shown with shaky and blurred camera work. In the end, he feels he is now transitioned into "second childlessness and mere oblivion."

McIntyre was also a salesman who was suddenly unable to work because of his stroke, and can now only utter one- to two-word sentences. The documentary has several interviews with speech therapists—some serious, some again mixed with attempts at humor. ("Look at this guy. He is Mr. Aphasia.") The film, made 6 years after his stroke, shows him with a marked expressive aphasia. It shows the marked devastation of aphasia in a person who used speech in his profession.

Picturing Aphasia is a film that shows several patients explaining their medical history—most after a stroke, some after a traumatic brain injury—which left them aphasic. The movie is impressive because it combines interview-style filming with the stories interpreted into a sequence of drawings (hence the title). This film was also made to raise awareness and understanding of aphasia, and it succeeds. The drawings provide visual symbols to improve communication. They help in understanding the spoken language and also emphasize how aphasia is perceived, and how patients with aphasia are disabled and cognitively impaired. The film also points to stigmatization and how difficult it is for patients when they cannot express themselves through words.

A Final Word

Aphasia may improve up to 6 months after a stroke, after which it reaches a plateau. Semantics and syntax may improve considerably up to 6 weeks; phonology and token test (measuring severity of aphasia) may improve up to 3 months. In patients with global aphasia, speech output may improve, but verbal communication lags behind.

To a certain degree, and depending on the severity of aphasia, outcome may be influenced by speech therapy. There is some evidence that early daily aphasia intervention improves communication, but recovery from aphasia due to a stroke remains variable and unpredictable. There are major interventions available for aphasia, such as melodic intonation and constraint-induced therapy—all of which are technology based. Current concepts focus on intertemporal lobe connectivity (with speech comprehension in the superior temporal cortex). Improvement was seen in aphasic patients who had such connectivity intact.

Aphasia has a significant effect on people's lives, and quality-of-life studies in stroke have not always studied the additional factors, including emotional distress and depression, the extent of aphasic impairment, the difficulty with communication, and productivity levels. There is also a marked variability of recovery from aphasia, and it appears that when improvement occurs, aphasia typically changes from a less severe form within the first year. This includes changing from nonfluent to fluent. Factors that play a consistent role in language recovery have not yet been identified.

Further Reading

Dobkin BH, Dorsch A. New evidence for therapies in stroke rehabilitation. *Curr Atheroscler Rep* 2013;15:331.

Hilari K, Needle JJ, Harrison KL. What are the important factors in health-related quality of life for people with aphasia? A systematic review. *Arch Phys Med Rehabil* 2012;93:S86–95.

Lazar RM, Antoniello D. Variability in recovery from aphasia. *Curr Neurol Neurosci Rep* 2008;8:497–502.

Warren JE, Crinion JT, Lambon Ralph MA, Wise RJ. Anterior temporal lobe connectivity correlates with functional outcome after aphasic stroke. *Brain* 2009;132:3428–42.

POLIOMYELITIS IN DOCUMENTARY FILM

A Paralyzing Fear: The Story of Polio in America (1998); directed by Nina Gilden Seavey, written by Stephan Chodorov and Nina Gilden Seavey; narrated by Olympia Dukakis; distributed by PBS Home Video.

Rating

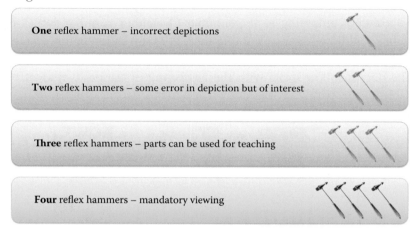

One reflex hammer – incorrect depictions

Two reflex hammers – some error in depiction but of interest

Three reflex hammers – parts can be used for teaching

Four reflex hammers – mandatory viewing

Criticism and Context

As mentioned in Chapter 3, poliomyelitis is mostly a disease of the past—at least in the developed world. *A Paralyzing Fear*—among other documentaries made over the years—is revealing because it touches on several major medical and sociologic themes. The documentary should be seen as a glimpse into summers in the early twentieth century that we really do not want to be reminded of. The firsthand experience of patients is troubling in this film and brings us back to a time when there was anxiety with every new summer. People were in fear that poliomyelitis ("the crippler") would strike. Patients would describe a "stiff neck, terrible pain, back pain, and every step I took would radiate through my body."

Quotable Lines of Dialogue

A Paralyzing Fear: The Story of Polio in America

Dr. Richard Aldrich	*We admitted 464 proven cases of polio just at the university hospital, which is unbelievable. And this was a very severe paralytic form. Maybe two or three hours after a lot of these kids would come in with a stiff neck or a fever, they'd be dead. It was unbelievable.*

The narration by Olympia Dukakis is serene and appropriate for the topic. The explanation of complex immunology is very well done and is simple and understandable. There were many fears and phobias. It was the fear of catching the disease, the fear of catching the worst kind, the fear of becoming ventilator dependent, fear of being exposed to complications of vaccinations, and the fear of the vaccine itself, which—at least in the early development stages—was actually responsible for several hundred cases of severe poliomyelitis. When a case of poliomyelitis occurred, panic was evident, with neighborhoods emptying in the summer ("neighbor running away from neighbor"), although to no avail (Figure 5.7). Many children, however, had only a mild form of the illness and were not affected by paralysis.

The documentary starts with the beginning of the polio epidemic in 1916. Infantile paralysis was known for many decades, but it was not

(a)

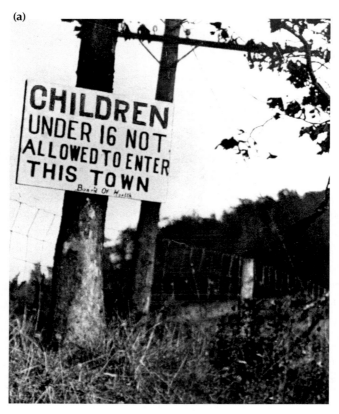

FIGURE 5.7　(a) Warning signs during the polio epidemic.

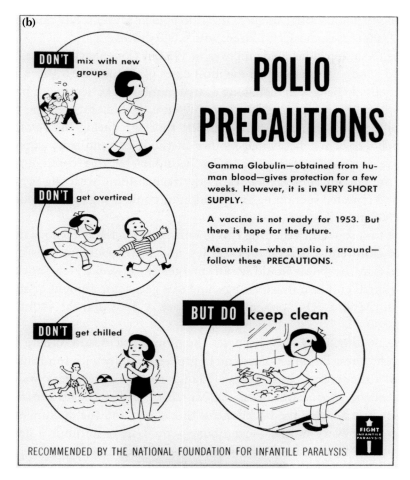

FIGURE 5.7 *(Continued)*   (b) A March of Dimes flyer distributed during the polio epidemic in the 1950s. (With permission of the March of Dimes.)

understood like other epidemics such as cholera and diphtheria. Many experts at the time felt that the 1916 epidemic was an aberrant event, and future upticks in infection "would never be as bad as this in the United States." The prevailing understanding was that it had to do with poor sanitation, and this resulted in one summer when officials killed hundreds of stray cats. Other sources were considered in New York City, and it did not take long for one to look at the slums and the newly arrived Italian and eastern European immigrants (see Chapter 3 on epidemic meningitis for a similar theme). The 1916 epidemic eventually numbered over 27,000 cases, mostly children, with 6,000 deaths.

The most notorious epidemic was in 1952 in Copenhagen, and in the United States, Minnesota had the most cases of all the states. There were enormous challenges in managing a large number of patients with poliomyelitis at the same time. Negative pressure ventilators were the only available ventilators, and their dramatic shortage during the zenith of the polio epidemic necessitated other methods of ventilatory support. Positive-pressure ventilation and tracheostomy became commonplace after the poliomyelitis epidemics. Early tracheostomy with bag ventilation and repeated suctioning and positioning could bring mortality down from 80% to 40%.

The first shock in watching this documentary is the enormous number of children in braces, on crutches, and in wheelchairs. It is mentioned that "hospitals would see an emergency for weeks." It is shocking to see small children in iron lungs, and this gets a fair amount of attention in the film. (One patient recalls a "sea of beds and the sounds of bellows.")

The documentary also discusses the humanistic desire to help others under these circumstances and to proceed rapidly with fundraising. "Small fundraising" was typical ("dance so that others may walk"), but a major effort came with the March of Dimes ("send a dime"). Housewives became the backbone of this effort, and the documentary shows that "every mother—even busy—could spare an hour a day to help out." Other creative ways were found to solicit money. At 7 p.m., sirens would go off and women would knock on doors to solicit for money. ("Turn on your porch light. Help fight polio tonight.") This charity raised millions.

The documentary also describes the academic struggles and cutthroat attitudes—the so-called Polio Wars—in some detail. The Salk (inactivated virus) vaccine would reduce the number of cases by 80% in 2 years, and even in 1955 the newspapers would declare the polio epidemic conquered, but then came the Cutter incident (referring to the Cutter Laboratories of Berkeley, California). Some lots of vaccine contained live virus and resulted in many infected children. In each case, paralysis occurred in the arm that was inoculated with a vaccine from Cutter Laboratories. The documentary does not mention that a jury found Cutter Laboratories not negligent but guilty of breaching an implied warranty. The Cutter incident reduced the willingness of pharmaceutical companies to make lifesaving vaccines.

The documentary also points to racial segregation in the South. Warm Springs in Georgia—the resort bought by Franklin D. Roosevelt to allow rehabilitation of polio patients—did not allow African Americans and necessitated a separate polio building in Tuskegee. The documentary does not address the (inaccurate) assumption at the time that African Americans were in some way immune to polio virus. It also shies away from the Kenny approach (Chapter 3) and presents her method of treating poliomyelitis as an incontrovertible fact. The documentary also does not discuss one of the major reasons polio is not eradicated in the developing world and the role that fundamentalist religious objections play there.

Another documentary on poliomyelitis, *The American Experience: The Polio Crusade* by Sarah Colt, aired on PBS in 2009. This documentary, well worth viewing, has much similar subject matter and is based on Oshinsky's Pulitzer Prize-winning book.

In addition to documentaries presenting a historical assessment of the polio epidemics in the United States, there are personal accounts. Two documentaries present polio survivors and their long-term care in an iron lung. One is a documentary by Jessica Yu, *Breathing Lessons: The Life and Work of Mark O'Brien* (1996), which is also a subject of the feature film *The Sessions* (2012), discussed in Chapter 3.

Martha Mason is the subject of another documentary film, *Martha in Lattimore* (2005) ✍. Lattimore is a small town with a population of not more than 400. Martha was 71 when she died, after living for more than 60 years in an iron lung. She chose to remain in an iron lung for the freedom it gave her, to avoid a tracheostomy and more complex care, and possible future hospitalizations. She could stay home, and the device took no professional skills to operate and was maintained by two aides. Martha bought a voice-activated computer that gave her access to e-mail and Internet browsing, and this technological advance furthered her ability to communicate. It also allowed her to write her memoir, *Breath: Life in the Rhythm of an Iron Lung*. She took care of her own affairs, paid bills, and even arranged for her mother's care when she became demented and aggressive.

Both of these biographical documentaries are somewhat disturbing. Why would patients stay in the iron lung so long when there are better and more efficient solutions? One can only speculate it may have to do with becoming psychologically attached to the machine. Many iron lungs were decorated with paint or decorative magnets, to give them personal touch. For many patients it is comfortable, and often these patients refused to be hospitalized unless the iron lung also came to the hospital when there was an intercurrent illness. Many patients simply felt that tracheostomy would kill them.

It is not known how many patients are still in an iron lung—the number it may approach 50 in the United States. Many patients would also use the so-called glossopharyngeal breathing—"frog" breathing. The technique was developed during the poliomyelitis epidemic. Patients used muscles of the mouth and pharynx to push air into the lower airways. Glossopharyngeal breathing has been an emergency method for patients confined to the iron lung, and this method could sustain ventilation for several hours.

A Final Word

The polio myelitis epidemic has been a major topic of scholarly work, and good insight into this neurologic disease can be obtained by watching these documentaries. Poliomyelitis remains a major problem in the underdeveloped world, where healthcare workers administering a polio vaccine are at risk (and some have been murdered). Poliomyelitis only flares up in regions where there is conflict and war and where there are religious objections. Elsewhere, poliomyelitis has largely been eradicated.

Further Reading

Kluger J. *Splendid Solution: Jonas Salk and the Conquest of Polio*. New York: Penguin, 2005.

Offit PA. *The Cutter Incident: How America's First Polio Vaccine Led to the Growing Vaccine Crisis*. New Haven, CN: Yale University Press, 2005.

Oshinsky DM. *Polio: An American Story*. Oxford, UK: Oxford University Press, 2005.

Shell M. *Polio and Its Aftermath: The Paralysis of Culture*. Cambridge, MA: Harvard University Press, 2005.

TRAUMATIC BRAIN INJURY IN FILM

The Crash Reel (2013); directed by Lucy Walker, written by Pedro Kos and Lucy Walker; distributed by HBO Films.

Rating

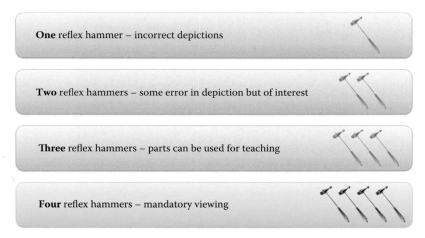

One reflex hammer – incorrect depictions

Two reflex hammers – some error in depiction but of interest

Three reflex hammers – parts can be used for teaching

Four reflex hammers – mandatory viewing

Criticism and Context

The Crash Reel is about snowboarder Kevin Pearce (Figure 5.8) and his major traumatic brain injury (TBI). The film shows Kevin through the use of a combination of home recordings and promotional videos highlighting his tremendous talents in half-pipe snowboarding, his development into stardom, and his competition with and outperformance of his major competitors.

The film opens with scenes of daredevil snowboarders and plenty of overconfidence. Kevin is explaining that a half-pipe with a 22-foot wall gives more "air time" and also provides "more tricks." He further adds that "people are going to be blown away with what they are going to see." This is during a training session in Park City, Utah, in 2009, about a month before the 2010 Winter Olympics.

Two days before the accident, the documentary shows a night of drinking. We later see Kevin trying out a new "cab double cork," which is a double backflip with a twist. He lands without sticking out his hands and with his face flat on the icy wall. He is immediately comatose, and a marked orbital hematoma is shown. Witnesses later tell us that he had to be intubated and was "shaking." Another bystander tells us that his left eye had a "blown pupil." He is helicoptered out into the neurointensive care unit, where he stays for 26 days. One of the first things the family hears about the accident—shown on film—is whether they could grant permission for a ventriculostomy. We get a glimpse of his MRI scan, which shows

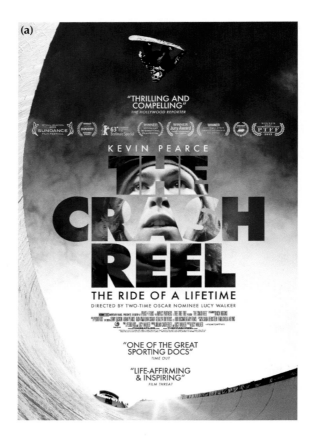

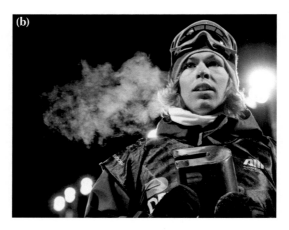

FIGURE 5.8 (a) Film poster of *The Crash Reel*; (b) Kevin Pearce (before his traumatic brain injury). (Used with permission from Prodigy Public Relations.)

multiple severe shearing lesions in the hippocampi and lesions peppered throughout the white matter. There is also a considerable intraventricular hemorrhage that likely prompted the ventriculostomy.

The documentary shows Kevin's slow recovery, and his brother explains the hospital course fairly well with his small incremental change, his inability to speak, Kevin's frustration ("constant new hurdles to get over"), and medical complications, including a deep venous thrombosis. Nothing seems to change in the first months, but then he begins to make large strides, or what his brother calls an "amazing ladder of a progression." While we see him improve, the documentary contrasts Kevin's situation with his competitor Shaun White earning a gold medal at the 2010 Vancouver Winter Olympics. Olympic medal contender Kevin Pearce, who was willing to push the boundaries to defeat Shaun White, has now deteriorated into a severely injured young man.

In an unprecedented way, the film shows the subtle but severe late consequences of TBI in elite athletes. Kevin takes antidepressants and two antiepileptic drugs and struggles with his memory and attention. He has episodes of confusion, impulsivity, and what he calls "sensory overload." There is also surgery to correct his double vision, and he has to wear corrective glasses. However, Kevin is unfazed and wants to start snowboarding again, and the film turns into a quite important moral lesson. His parents feel understandable guilt that they did not stop Kevin from engaging in such a high-risk sport and that they gradually got caught up in the "branding and selling" of their son.

Quotable Lines of Dialogue

The Crash Reel	
Mother	*I was so surprised they do see people with a second one [TBI] and a third one.... I thought if someone had one, why would they put themselves in a situation where they might have another one?*
Kevin	*It's really hard for you guys to know. It is unexplainable.... I just feel like no one else in this room has that feeling about anything.*

The documentary shows multiple conversations around the kitchen table, with family members trying to discourage Kevin from going back to snowboarding. Kevin bluntly tells them that he feels that "there is no trust" in his family, and his father counters that he puts his family at risk. It is clear that his family feels that it is not fair to ask them to take care of him should there be another injury. Kevin eventually tries snowboarding, but it becomes clear that he has lost his confidence and no longer has the coordination for the sport. Most of the documentary shows him becoming aware of this defeat.

There is a delicate boundary over which it is hard to step. Athletes may want to go back after an injury, but very few, have succeeded in elite sports. Kevin became a motivational speaker and a compassionate advocate for TBI (on his website you can buy his LoveYourBrain T-shirts).

This documentary offers a unique window into the significance of injuries associated with these types of extreme sports. Some athletes have more severe injury or death, such as Sarah Burke, a world champion freestyle skier, who died as a result of a traumatic head injury sustained during a practice run—in the same half-pipe where Kevin Pearce had his injury. She is mentioned here too, and the documentary briefly touches on the substantial medical costs as a result of injury. It is suggested that Sarah Burke was not insured, and her sponsors would only pay for her medical costs if accidents occurred during events. (Her costs eventually were covered through fundraising efforts.)

This documentary is a unique example of the rehabilitation of traumatic head injury and its long-term effects, particularly in young individuals who physically seem to have completely recovered. It shows the unstoppable drive to return to their original athletic prowess, only to find that it is no longer possible. It also emphasizes that, not surprisingly, these accidents can be fatal, and that a devastating traumatic injury can take place in a split second. For the youngsters who survive, the hospital course is endless, and the film shows the complexity of care with rehabilitation physicians, psychiatrists, and ophthalmologists, who all are involved with Kevin's care.

Injuries among snowboarders are more frequent (two to three times higher) than in skiers; improper landing from high amplitude jumps is the most common mechanism for elite snowboarders. Studies have reported head and face injury in approximately 1 of 10 elite snowboarders. In addition, more than 1 in 4 skiers and snowboarders are at risk of a major traumatic head injury by not wearing a helmet or wearing an insufficient helmet. Snowboarders and skiers have a tendency to wear ski hats below their helmets, causing improper fit and risk of displacement during sudden acceleration-deceleration impact.

The documentary touches on the well-publicized so-called second-impact syndrome. Usually this controversial syndrome occurs soon after the incident while the patient is still symptomatic. The first minor concussion is followed by rapid fatal coma from brain swelling during the "second" impact. The main mechanism is impaired autoregulation of cerebral blood flow, with the first blow allowing massive cerebral edema and increased intracranial pressure after the second blow. The existence of second-impact syndrome has been accepted, but it is likely very rare and is seen shortly after a first injury.

The film is also about recovery and recovery potential, showing other injured teenagers and optimistic rehabilitation physicians. ("He is going to get a lot better. Come see him in a year."). It may be farfetched to compare Kevin's brain injuries with other brain injuries ("your brain looks so much better than this guy"—referring to an NFL running back's MRI, which was likely affected with chronic traumatic encephalopathy). Kevin's injury should be set apart from chronic traumatic encephalopathy—a neurodegenerative disorder showing diffuse accumulation of hyperphosphorylated tau. This disorder, in the past mostly connected to boxing ("punch drunk"), has been correlated with out-of-control, explosive, verbal, violent behaviors, but the risks are not yet well defined and are possibly exaggerated, and the feared parkinsonism may not be present in many patients. Chronic traumatic encephalopathy injury should also be set apart from "concussions," defined by the American Academy of Neurology as grade 1: transient confusion resolving in 15 minutes ("the bell ringer"); grade 2: longer-lasting symptoms of transient confusion but no unconsciousness; and grade 3: a concussion with loss of consciousness.

A Final Word

Traumatic head injury in freestyle skiers and snowboarders is not uncommon, and 10% of the 2,080 injuries during seven World Cup seasons were due to contusions (two were fatal). Some sports, such as half-pipe and snowboard cross, may be just too dangerous. Using new tricks and pushing the limits is necessary to win, and the winners are those snowboarders who are able to flip in three different planes. In Sochi 2014, Iouri Podladtchikov (also known as iPod) won with his impressive flip called the YOLO (You Only Live Once).

In addition, gear technology may have difficulty catching up with the major "advances" in highly competitive sports. Although helmets are compulsory, helmet standards are constantly changing, and there is active research in video analysis of injuries. There are also other pressing questions: Are the goggles, which improve peripheral vision but reduce skull protection, too big? Are face-protection helmets needed, and how "uncool" is that? There are no answers to these serious concerns about where this elite sport is going. *The Crash Reel* confronts all of these questions but also has many other subtexts. It is an astounding documentary about recovery of traumatic head injury in young athletes. The film is unique and important in showing the gradual and steady improvement of young individuals recovering from a TBI. It also shows what families have to face. The tremendous duress of the parents is obvious and is portrayed well. What do parents do with a child who now has a major handicap and lack of insight as a result of the brain injury? Kevin's father says that an e-mail he received told him that "you need to be prepared for the Kevin who comes back not to be the same Kevin."

Further Reading

Cantu RC. Second-impact syndrome. *Clin Sports Med* 1998;17:37–44.

Cundy TP, Systermans BJ, Cundy WJ, et al. Helmets for snow sports: Prevalence, trends, predictors and attitudes to use. *J Trauma* 2010;69:1486–90.

Klein AM, Howell K, Vogler J, et al. Rehabilitation outcome of unconscious traumatic brain injury patients. *J Neurotrauma* 2013;30:1476–83.

Levy AS, Hawkes AP, Hemminger LM, Knight S. An analysis of head injuries among skiers and snowboarders. *J Trauma* 2002;53:695–704.

McKee AC, Stern RA, Nowinski CJ, et al. The spectrum of disease in chronic traumatic encephalopathy. *Brain* 2013;136:43–64.

Meehan WP, 3rd, Bachur RG. Sport-related concussion. *Pediatrics* 2009;123:114–23.

Quality Standards Subcommittee. Practice parameter: The management of concussion in sports (summary statement). Report of the Quality Standards Subcommittee. *Neurology* 1997;48:581–85.

Steenstrup SE, Bere T, Bahr R. Head injuries among FIS World Cup alpine and freestyle skiers and snowboarders: A 7-year cohort study. *Br J Sports Med* 2014;48:41–45.

Wetjen NM, Pichelmann MA, Atkinson JL. Second impact syndrome: Concussion and second injury brain complications. *J Am Coll Surg* 2010;211:553–57.

Wijdicks CA, Rosenbach BS, Flanagan TR, et al. Injuries in elite and recreational snowboarders. *Br J Sports Med* 2014;48:11–17.

Zemper ED. Two-year prospective study of relative risk of a second cerebral concussion. *Am J Phys Med Rehabil* 2003;82:653–59.

REHABILITATION IN FILM

Coma (2007); directed by Liz Garbus; distributed by Moxie Firecracker Films and HBO Documentaries.

Rating

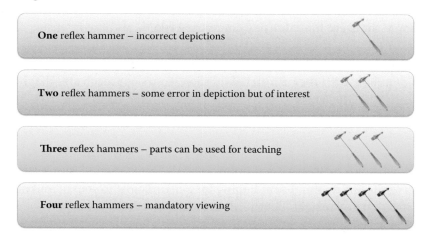

One reflex hammer – incorrect depictions

Two reflex hammers – some error in depiction but of interest

Three reflex hammers – parts can be used for teaching

Four reflex hammers – mandatory viewing

Criticism and Context

Documentaries on rehabilitation in coma are virtually nonexistent. Filmed over the course of one year, *Coma* profiles four young patients with catastrophic traumatic head injury who were treated at the Center for Head Injuries at the JFK Medical Center in Edison, New Jersey. Though better than previous media portrayals of this topic, the documentary has shortcomings. The film shows hopeful families and friends deeply and compassionately involved with the care of their loved one, but the uncensored surreal abundance of pity, sorrow, and loneliness that continues for more than 100 unrelenting minutes makes the film hard to watch. Another problem is the title. Eventually, three of the four patients emerge from what appears to be a coma. Perhaps a more appropriate, although less appealing, title would be "Coping with a Catastrophic Head Trauma." Another issue is that the mise-en-scène is essentially in the neurorehabilitation center. This would normally be an unlikely setting because most centers see only a small proportion of patients with catastrophic neurologic injury. In fact, only patients who have recovered qualify for a rehabilitation program.

The film starts with the statement, "The mystery of coma and brain injury has captivated America's imagination for decades." This is followed by snippets of newspaper and magazine articles, such as "What if something is going on in there?" "Twilight Zone," and with Senate leader and cardiovascular surgeon Bill Frist declaring that a minimally conscious state is "a tough diagnosis to make." The director primes us to believe that with prolonged comatose states, there is an ominous uncertainty. The use of the Terri Schiavo case is unclear, and this movie is not about her.

Some shots are filmed inside conference rooms and the intensive care unit. In allowing filming here, the staff and family open themselves up for scrutiny, including clever montages, camera angles, and close-ups. One could quibble with the neurorehabilitation team's approach and diagnostic accuracy. Their task is never easy. There is often confusion. Nowhere is this more evident than in a scene showing elated parents when they are told their son is not in a minimally conscious state. Next they are told that word deafness is a major contributor to his condition. To see them recoil when his neurologic condition, after all, is not so good is unsettling. During the entire film, I kept hoping for a neurologist to step in and offer clarification and insight, but this doesn't happen.

Quotable Lines of Dialogue

Coma	
Father	*I do not know what is the worst thing you want your doctor to say, but you hear it all the time, "Sean is unique; Sean is an enigma."*
Father	*I asked myself repeatedly, "What were these families told? Why the overwhelming incredulity and ambiguity? What were their expectations in the first place? Was there denial?"*

The director punctuates these heartrending stories with segments of unbridled optimism and with an atmosphere where healthcare providers are mired in a feeling of uncertainty ("All brain injuries are different"). At the end of the documentary, we see one of the families providing home care for their son, who is in a permanent vegetative state. Disturbingly, the mother tries to spoon-feed him, which is a highly dangerous maneuver for a person in this state.

So, I thought, "What would I like to see in a documentary, and what would best serve the public?" At the risk of being presumptuous, I would like to see a documentary show the entire spectrum of recovery from coma in intensive care units to neurorehabilitation centers. Patients typically become comatose from devastating traumatic brain injury, aneurysmal subarachnoid hemorrhage, fulminant encephalitis, or anoxic-ischemic injury after cardiopulmonary resuscitation.

Withdrawal of life support in patients who fail to awaken is not an uncommon outcome, often prompted by advance directives but also after extensive deliberation about realistic outcomes with family members. Coverage of such a family conference would show the complexity of these conversations. Perhaps such a documentary could also show the benefits of organ and tissue donation after a comatose patient becomes brain dead, and the relief it could provide for many families. A documentary should also emphasize the wide range of possible outcomes from a catastrophic brain injury, including the promises and limitations of neurorehabilitation.

Most comatose patients and those in a minimally conscious state are cared for in a nursing home, but there are uniquely specialized centers, such as the JFK Medical Center, that admit patients for care and research. Disorders of consciousness, particularly when severe or prolonged, are artificially divided into minimally conscious state and persistent vegetative state, and physicians use several clinical tools to differentiate between the two (Table 5.1). For families, to make that distinction is difficult, and there are always moments when they think they see "more responsiveness." For physicians, the challenge is to judge these reactions accurately and not to easily dismiss them as "reflexes." Unfortunately, there are too many instances in which the physician has ignored families' observations, and when the patient improves there is much consternation and distrust. Prolonged observation by multiple healthcare providers skilled in this work is the only way to ascertain lack of awareness or improvement in responsiveness.

A Final Word

For the public, *Coma* is an unprecedented look at the composure of some families suddenly struck with a disaster but who see a silver lining in the dark cloud. In depicting a bleak outcome for some patients, the director

TABLE 5.1 Distinguishing Clinical Features between Persistent Vegetative State (PVS) and Minimally Conscious State (MCS)

Test	PVS	MCS
Eyes	Not tracking a finger	Tracking or fixating
Verbal	Absent	Sounds
		Moans
		Words
Grimacing	Absent (mostly)	Present
Sounds	Startle	Looks to sound
Movement	Reflex only	Purposeful

gets her point across. It is less useful for students of medicine and nursing as well as healthcare providers. The director's suggestion that patients who have a slow recovery are allowed to have prolonged lengths of stay in rehabilitation centers is inaccurate. In addition, this documentary does not elaborate on current ethical, legal, and financial issues. I struggled to identify the purpose of this documentary because it is without context. Nothing here explains coma. The film does not address (a) the diagnostic certainty that exists in many instances based on the well-known prognostic indicators or (b) the questionable effect of pharmacologic interventions or so-called stimulation programs and the speculative nature of many of the newly introduced therapies. Rehabilitation physicians are divided on how to approach these unfortunate patients.

Further Reading

Bernat JL. Chronic disorders of consciousness. *Lancet* 2006;367:1181–92.

Giacino JT, Katz DI, Whyte J. Neurorehabilitation in disorders of consciousness. *Semin Neurol* 2013;33:142–56.

Giacino J, Whyte J. The vegetative and minimally conscious states: Current knowledge and remaining questions. *J Head Trauma Rehabil* 2005;20:30–50.

Lee TM, Savage J, McKee H, et al. How do you know when your patient is "waking up": Coma recovery assessment in a complex continuing care setting. *Can J Neurosci Nurs* 2013;35:27–33.

Wijdicks EFM. *The Comatose Patient*. 2nd ed. Oxford, UK: Oxford University Press, 2014.

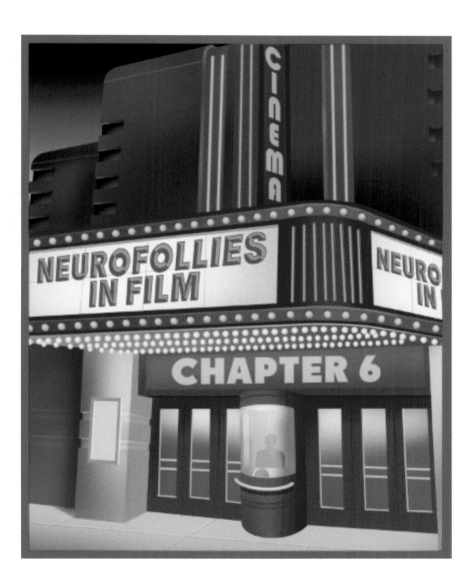

CHAPTER **6**

Neurofollies in Film

Hall 9000: ...This conversation can serve no purpose anymore, goodbye.

2001:A Space Odyssey (1968)

INTRODUCING MAIN THEMES

One could question whether medicine (doctors and diseases) is an appropriate topic for entertainment, but that has not stopped screenwriters. In fact, screenplays may be more interesting when there is creative exaggeration and silliness. The renowned filmmaker Jean-Luc Godard famously said, "Cinema is the most beautiful fraud in the world." Some may protest this contention, but isn't it ironic that inaccurate and absurd films are sometimes also the most loved?

There is a considerable amount of neurologic nonsense in horror movies involving the brain (*The Brain Eaters* [1958], *Brain Damage* [1988], *The Brain That Wouldn't Die* [1962]), but these films are a particular genre. There is a renewed interest in zombie and vampire themes, but none are specifically related to neurologic conditions; these are more related to life after death.

Some films in this category are classic comedies (*The Man with Two Brains* [1983] featuring Steve Martin), while others may just have a single "funny" scene. The John Landis-directed, groundbreaking slapstick *Kentucky Fried Movie* (1977) has a scene in a "headache research center." Patients are shown with their heads being slammed against the wall, hit by reflex hammers, and struck with glass bottles—all to test the painkiller "Sanhedrin Extra Strength."

Some films use neurologic injury to give the villain an advantage, such as *The World Is Not Enough* (1999). In this film, the villain, a KGB agent turned terrorist, has a bullet through the medulla oblongata "killing off his senses" and now is able to "push himself harder than any normal man."

Neurologic absurdity also extends into science fiction. Mind control, brain stimulation, "entering" the mind, and other far-out stories interest screenwriters. A larger perceptive analysis on science fiction and neurology yet has to be written. Curiously, films dealing with futuristic neurology may actually seem very real, and that is were the interest lies.

The main purpose of this chapter is to discuss films with potential plausibility and to explore where these fantastical ideas could have come from. In this chapter, ten remarkable films are rated—be warned it is all cockamamie. One could argue that a critical review of neurofollies may not serve a purpose. The artistic control of filmmakers will not change; film makers often purposely satirize a plot and thus if it is leads to pure cinema, who wants to quibble with that?

ENTER THE MIND

The Cell (2000); starring Jennifer Lopez, Vince Vaughn, and Vincent D'Onofrio; directed by Tarsem Singh, written by Mark Protosevich; distributed by New Line Cinema.

Rating

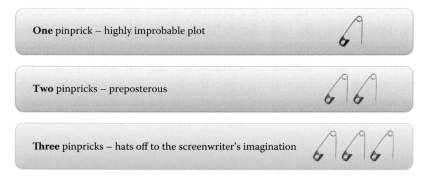

One pinprick – highly improbable plot

Two pinpricks – preposterous

Three pinpricks – hats off to the screenwriter's imagination

Criticism and Context

The Cell suggests that there may be future techniques that could have one person enter the mind of another. This film is a complex thriller that involves a schizophrenic killer named Stargher (Vincent D'Onofrio) who lapses into a catatonic state after a recent crime. This occurs after he notices he is being trailed by the FBI. (To be fair, we see a very good representation of catatonia here, with what appears to be a rigid composure, a fixed gaze, shivering, and sweating.)

Without giving away too much of the plot, it becomes clear to the investigators that the only way to solve the main character's crime is to enter his mind. Using sophisticated technology ("Neuromed") the child psychologist Catherine Deane (Jennifer Lopez) is able to do so. The film is cinematically spectacular, and scenes show Stargher's early memories and traumas as a child as well as fantastical gothic worlds. The film suggests that our memories are simply boxed-in stories that we can access. The film shows that the brain of this psychopathic killer is full of violent vivid scenery and is simmering with anger.

The "Neuromed" technology shown in this film will immediately remind neurologists of a functional MRI, and the "Neuromed" seems like the next advancement in MRI technology. There is no question that MRI technology has made a major contribution to our understanding of brain activity; it has already demonstrated that certain brain areas become activated by motor tasks and emotions. In recent studies of unresponsive patients, communication has been established through complex pathways in one or two patients, but there is not yet a reproducible way of doing that. For many rehabilitation physicians, it is unclear whether a consistent response can be generated that would allow a brain–computer interface to function.

Given everything else, this film shows how to use a device to "communicate" with unresponsive patients and may have a kernel of truth. To "enter" a mind is unfathomable.

PSYCHIC AFTER COMA

The Dead Zone (1983); starring Christopher Walken, Brooke Adams, and Tom Skerritt; directed by David Cronenberg, written by Stephen King (adapted novel) and Jeffrey Boam; distributed by Paramount Pictures.

Rating

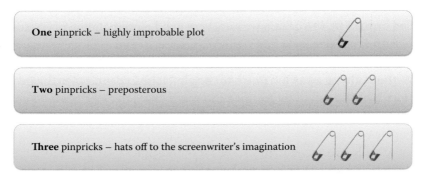

One pinprick – highly improbable plot

Two pinpricks – preposterous

Three pinpricks – hats off to the screenwriter's imagination

Criticism and Context

The Dead Zone is adapted from a novel by Stephen King. The protagonist Johnny (played by Christopher Walken) wakes up in a skilled nursing facility. His physician Dr. Weizak explains that he has been in a motor vehicle accident. ("You have been our guest here for a while.") Johnny looks confused and finds he has no bandages or visible injury, and asks why he is in here. His parents are brought in, and they tell Johnny that he has been in a coma for 5 years. ("The Lord has delivered you from your trance.") Dr. Weizak, visibly irritated, corrects them, "No, he has been in a coma, not in a trance." Dr. Weizak is the rehabilitation physician who tells him, "Your therapy will be long and painful, but you will walk."

Johnny discovers he has "extrasensory perception." When he touches a nurse, he has a vision that her daughter is in a fire. (This turns out to be true, and she is saved as a result of his vision.) When he touches Dr. Weizak, Johnny has a vision of violent World War II scenes of people fleeing Poland. (Johnny tells Doctor Weizak his mother is still alive, and it turns out that this, too, is true.) It is now clear that Johnny has become psychic. He cannot only see the future, but can also change it by altering events. These premonitory signs are a major plot line in the movie.

The viewer may not need convincing evidence to show that there is no such thing as premonitions after a severe traumatic brain head injury (and certainly not after being in a 5-year vegetative state). However, severe traumatic brain injury leading to prolonged coma may be followed by a posttraumatic stress disorder that may involve night terrors. Receiving visions (or even a sense of coming doom) is not a manifestation of severe brain injury. However, it may fit with the general idea that personalities can change after a traumatic brain injury—and why not for the good? A similar theme arises in the film *Regarding Henry* (Chapter 3).

The Dead Zone is emblematic of Cronenberg's catalog of films with hallucinatory surreal worlds, and it remains a classic Stephen King novel. Recovery from a vegetative state is not common. It is virtually impossible after 5 years, and patients lack cognitive abilities, including precognition.

TOTAL AMNESIA

50 First Dates (2004); starring Adam Sandler, Drew Barrymore, Rob Schneider, and Dan Aykroyd; directed by Peter Segal, written by George Wing; distributed by Columbia Pictures.

Rating

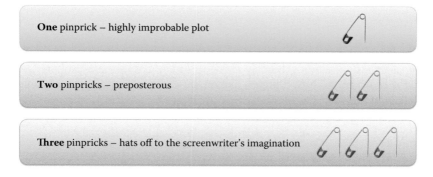

One pinprick – highly improbable plot

Two pinpricks – preposterous

Three pinpricks – hats off to the screenwriter's imagination

Criticism and Context

In *50 First Dates*, Lucy (Drew Barrymore), after a motor vehicle accident, forgets every day or, as her family friend says, "It's like her slate gets wiped clean every time she sleeps." The film is a screwball comedy. Every day Lucy wakes up thinking it is October 13—the day of the accident—and all of her days are similar. The whole family plays along. Eventually she discovers, by seeing a newspaper with a different date, that she has been deceived. She sees a neurologist (Dan Aykroyd), who tells her that the condition is known as the "Goldfield Syndrome," described by a brilliant Lithuanian psychiatrist. With this syndrome, she is unable to convert short-term memory into long-term memory. The neurologist points to her parietal lobe and proclaims, "I see that your sense of humor is intact. You have a magnificent amygdala as well."

Because Lucy's memory loss is such a surprise and major disappointment for her, the neurologist introduces her to "Ten-Second Tom," who apparently forgets everything every 10 seconds, and in one scene is seen constantly introducing himself to others.

There is some truth to the existence of this type of amnesic syndrome, and it reminds us of the film *Memento* (2000). There is a detailed discussion on this type of amnesic syndrome in Chapter 3.

A similar theme is shown in *Clean Slate* (1994), where the protagonist has no problems with his memory during wakefulness but loses his memories during sleep. Inability to memorize is well known, but losing all memories during sleep is not.

Another noteworthy movie is *Groundhog Day* (1990), in which all of the actors forget prior events, allowing the leading character (played brilliantly by Bill Murray) to correct—and that is the point—his blunders in courting his colleague.

ENHANCING BRAIN FUNCTION

Limitless (2011); starring Bradley Cooper, Abbie Cornish, and Robert De Niro; directed by Neil Burger, written by Leslie Dixon; distributed by Relativity Media.

Rating

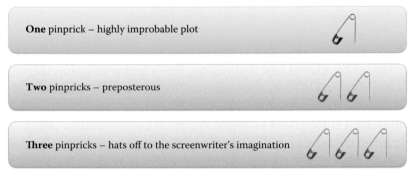

One pinprick – highly improbable plot

Two pinpricks – preposterous

Three pinpricks – hats off to the screenwriter's imagination

Criticism and Context

In *Limitless*, the leading character Eddie (played by Bradley Cooper) has writer's block and is told that there is a pill that can improve his brain function. It is stated here that "typically we only access 20% of our brain" and that Eddie's brain will work much better if he would only take a small, colorless pill that contains a neurostimulant. When he does, his senses drastically improve, and this is cleverly depicted by suddenly changing the scene hues from dark-blue into gold-yellow. His eyes now have a light-blue color. He starts writing his book. The neurotropic drug is called NZT48. Eddie also uses his dramatically improved brain function to play the stock market and become wealthy.

The film poses an interesting question regarding whether drugs may be developed that can improve brain function, assuming that there are dormant areas (apparently 80% according to this script) that need to be stimulated. The unfortunate fact is that no drug can do this. Many stimulants (amphetamines, cocaine, and ecstasy) change the senses temporarily, but none improve productivity, artistic ability, or intelligence. Similar statements have been made about alcohol and writers, but there is no evidence that there has ever been a positive effect. Stimulants have major side effects, including hallucinations and behavioral changes, and the sad truth is that drug use by artists (writers, composers, actors) often leads to serious addiction and sometimes death. This theme—how much of the brain we use—interests screenwriters. According to them it may not amount to much, and it is even less in a more recent film. In *Lucy* (2014) the active part of the brain is set at 10% (neurons may indeed take up only 10%, but guess what? We use 100% of the brain most of the time.)

INTELLECTUAL DISABILITY TO GENIUS

Charly (1968); starring Cliff Robertson, Claire Bloom, and Leon Janney; directed by Ralph Nelson, written by Stirling Silliphant; Academy Award for best actor (Cliff Robertson); distributed by Cinerama.

Rating

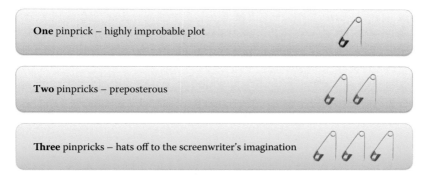

One pinprick – highly improbable plot

Two pinpricks – preposterous

Three pinpricks – hats off to the screenwriter's imagination

Criticism and Context

The starring role is Charly, played by Cliff Robertson. He has a disability: an IQ of only 59 ("retardate"), and at his work he is often the butt of jokes. Testing shows that he has difficulty writing and often writes in mirror images. (He writes his name as CHAЯLY). When Charly is subjected to a maze test identical to one traversed by a mouse, the mouse beats him consistently.

Charly wants to be smarter and he undergoes (unspecified) brain surgery from which he gradually improves. He becomes highly intelligent and suddenly has a good grasp of abstract theoretical metaphysics. His IQ now approaches genius category. He is now also serious marriage material and develops a relationship with his prior schoolteacher, Alice Kinian (played by Claire Bloom), but emotionally he remains a child. Unfortunately, his intelligence fades, and as a result of this decisive turn he is unable to marry Alice—even when she insists. The film ends on a sad note. The movie *Charly* was adapted from the novel *Flowers for Algernon* (the name of the mouse).

It is difficult to grasp why (in the 1960s) brain surgery was suggested to improve intelligence. The film is more about the limitations of living with a disability and being out of reach, which may have explained its success. It is remarkable that the film was apparently approved by the Presidential Committee for Mental Retardation.

SUPERINTELLIGENCE

Phenomenon (1996); starring John Travolta, Kyra Sedgwick, and Robert Duvall; directed by Jon Turteltaub, written by Gerald Di Pego; distributed by Buena Vista Pictures.

Rating

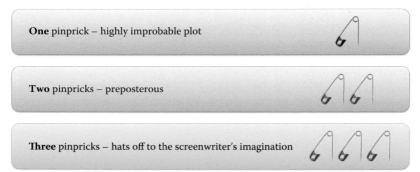

One pinprick – highly improbable plot

Two pinpricks – preposterous

Three pinpricks – hats off to the screenwriter's imagination

Criticism and Context

Phenomenon is about George Malley (John Travolta), who while looking up sees a bright light coming out of the sky that knocks him unconscious. This is a life-changing event. He now reads more than two books a day, complex crossword puzzles are a breeze, and everything seems "clearer" to him. But there is more, and George now "feels" pre-earthquake activity and develops levitation and telekinetic abilities. With his super intelligence, he is able to decode top-secret code signals. The film becomes even more preposterous when his unusual symptomatology is found to be due to a brain tumor, and this comes as a surprise at the end of the film. Apparently, this malignant astrocytoma does not cause a defect, but in fact, due to its "tentacles," stimulates parts of the brain. This gets the attention of the medical community, and he is admitted for observation. One neurosurgeon suggests performing awake surgery "to understand his brain better," and he hopes he will be "science's greatest teacher." When George realizes that this surgery is likely fatal and may be a ploy, he escapes. He dies suddenly and peacefully in the arms of his lover, with his last words being "It's happening." The film represents a gross misrepresentation of progression of a malignant brain tumor. The film also grossly misrepresents medical science and suggests there is an inclination of neurosurgeons to experiment on unusual cases (Chapter 4).

VIOLENT SEIZURES

The Terminal Man (1974); starring George Segal, Joan Hackett, Richard Dysart, and Jill Clayburgh; directed by Mike Hodges, written by Michael Crichton and Mike Hodges; distributed by Warner Bros.

Rating

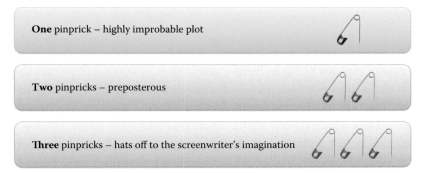

One pinprick – highly improbable plot

Two pinpricks – preposterous

Three pinpricks – hats off to the screenwriter's imagination

Criticism and Context

The Terminal Man is adapted from a novel by Michael Crichton, who also wrote *Coma* (1978), a film about organ trafficking. This film starts with a discussion at the dinner table between psychiatrists and neurosurgeons about a new operation for violent seizures. The surgery has been tried in animals, but Harry Benson (played by George Segal) will be the first human, and the surgeons will use electrode implantation to electrically control the seizures. He has violent seizures of which he has no recollection. One of the physicians says, "Nobody thinks of these people as physically ill. They are predisposed to violence, aggressive behavior, hypersexuality, pathological intoxication." Apparently, because Harry has uncontrollable rages but not physical seizures, the decision is made to stimulate the structures of the limbic system (involved with emotion and behavior) and to proceed with "limbic brain pacing." A computer will be connected to these grids that can fully control these seizures.

Before the surgery, the patient and treatment proposal are presented in a conference to a group of physicians, but one of the physicians stands up and starts to rail against psychosurgery and the wrongs that lobotomy has done. (It is explained to him that this is not a lobotomy.) Harry undergoes awake stereotactic operation. In the postoperative phase, each of the electrodes is stimulated, causing different sensations each time. One stimulus makes him feel that he has eaten ham sandwiches; another one causes an urge to urinate. Stimulation of yet another electrode causes uncontrollable laughing. Another stimulation has him make sexual advances to the investigator, and one stimulated electrode makes him behave "like a 5-year-old." When he describes his aura, he says he smells "pig shit and turpentine." He further describes the seizure as being angry and being on a rollercoaster that he cannot stop. ("There is no feeling like that in the world.") Initially, treatment seems successful, but then seizures return and are even more severe than before. Eventually the seizures take control, and he starts killing, which is preceded by a spell which is shown as eyes turning up and an angry grimace.

There is no such thing as limbic stimulation or control of seizures with implanted electrodes that, when stimulated, cause very specific responses. Where the film touches on reality is with a partly accurate description of temporal lobe epilepsy, and the literature on violence in temporal lobe epilepsy is abundant. Most neurologists have seen postictal violence or violent automatism. However, it should be pointed out that there have been very few acquittals of persons with epilepsy on the basis of criminal insanity, and murder as a result of temporal lobe epilepsy has not been proven. (Also see Chapter 3 on violent sleepwalking.) The film may also refer to the Klüver–Bucy syndrome, which may develop after a right temporal lobectomy to treat epilepsy and is characterized by hyperphagia and hypersexuality.

All the elements are here, and they superficially mimic the current state of treatment of intractable seizures (i.e., a vagal nerve stimulator), but in the end it does not add up. This is one example where it all seems deceptively real. If asked about the film, neurologists, epileptologists, or neurosurgeons would have a lot of explaining to do.

COMPUTER-ASSISTED NEURONAL ACTIVITY

BrainWaves (1983); starring Tony Curtis, Keir Dullea, Suzanna Love, and Vera Miles; directed by Ulli Lommel; distributed by MGM Studios.

Rating

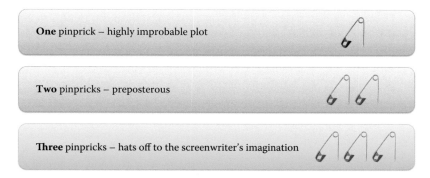

One pinprick – highly improbable plot

Two pinpricks – preposterous

Three pinpricks – hats off to the screenwriter's imagination

Criticism and Context

The theme of the science fiction movie *BrainWaves* is the replacement of defective areas of the brain with new brain activity. The head neuroscientist is Dr. Clavius (Tony Curtis), who uses fresh corpses to extract neuronal activity from the brain into a computer. (The assumption here is that although the body is dead, the brain still has electric activity.)

This is how it works. First, Dr. Clavius maps the brain of a comatose patient and identifies the "defective areas." He then uses this map to replace damaged neuronal activity with new electrical activity he has previously stored on a computer, as if he is putting replacement parts in. Everyone in the film seems impressed. There is a discussion in which one of the neurosurgeons remarks about this neuroscientist, "Dr. Clavius's methods can be unusual, but his work and his results are extraordinary."

The film shows a traffic accident that puts the leading female character into a coma. In an effort to help her regain consciousness, Dr. Clavius—looking deadly serious—wants to awaken her with the neuronal pattern of someone else. The film shows her brain "fed" with brainwaves, and she awakens and gradually recovers all function. However, then she has night terrors, and now it appears that she has been given the "neuronal pattern" of a young girl who was murdered. She not only sees images of this girl's murder but eventually is able to recognize the identity of the girl's killer.

This film suggests that not only can EEG activity be captured, stored, and transplanted, but also that EEG represents thought and memory. There is not a sliver of accuracy in this dark film. (The neuroscientist is not so friendly either.)

MIND CONTROL

Donovan's Brain (1953); starring Lew Ayres, Gene Evans, Nancy Davis Reagan, and Steve Brodie; directed by Felix Feist, written by Curt Siodmak (adapted novel) and Hugh Brooke; distributed by United Artists.

Rating

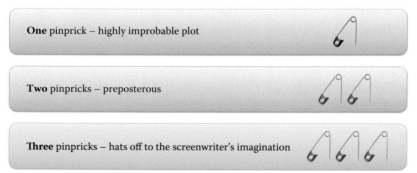

One pinprick – highly improbable plot

Two pinpricks – preposterous

Three pinpricks – hats off to the screenwriter's imagination

Criticism and Context

One of the cult classics in science fiction is *Donovan's Brain*. Dr. Cory (Lew Ayres) experiments with monkey brains by placing them in solutions, sticking in electrodes, registering brain waves, and imaging these with an oscillo-graph. When he is called to assess a plane accident, he steals the brain of a well-known businessman. He preserves the brain of this millionaire—unbe-knownst to him the man had prior shady dealings—in a way similar to his work with monkeys. Electrodes pick up activity, and the brain is seen glowing and pulsating. ("It looks like a beta frequency…oh it is…the brain must be thinking systematically.") Through telepathy—and here it becomes even more dicey—"the brain" makes Dr. Cory act out the businessman's bad thoughts.

Of course this has to stop, and in the final scene, "the brain" gets shot—but to no avail—and only after connecting the brain with electrical wires to a lightning rod during a storm is "the brain" destroyed, burning to pieces.

Dr. Cory is saved and confesses that things got out of hand. It is sug-gested that he may even survive a medical board examination into his ethics. If that would happen, he contemplates he might come back as a "country doctor," to which his wife (Nancy Reagan) responds, "No, dear, you are a scientist and always will be."

BRAIN PRESERVATION

The Brain That Wouldn't Die (1959); starring Jason Evers, Virginia Leith, and Eddie Carmel; directed by Joseph Green, written by Rex Carlton and Joseph Green; distributed by American International Pictures.

Rating

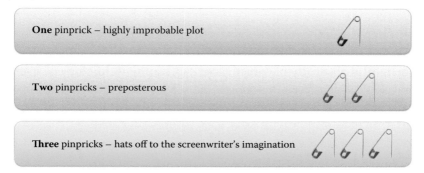

One pinprick – highly improbable plot

Two pinpricks – preposterous

Three pinpricks – hats off to the screenwriter's imagination

Criticism and Context

The Brain That Wouldn't Die is about bringing the dead back to life, and preserving a full head. In this film, Dr. Cortner (Jason Evers) is a plastic surgeon who experiments with transplantation in his (why not?) country home. The film opens with an operation performed by father and son, but the patient unfortunately dies on the table. The son asks his father if he can do an experiment because, really, "He is dead; I cannot do any harm." His father agrees. "Very well, the corpse is yours. Do what you want to do." Dr. Cortner stimulates the brain with electrodes while his father performs open heart massage that brings the patient back. Despite this success, the father warns, "The line between scientific genius and obsessive fanaticism is a thin line."

In the next scene, we see Dr. Cortner driving his car with his wife, Jane Compton (Virginia Leith). The car careens into a ditch and the wife is decapitated. He runs away with her head, and upon arrival at his country home/research laboratory, he connects her head to several tubes. She remains fully awake, although her voice is a bit hoarse. The film ends with him trying to drug a model and to connect her perfect body to his wife, but he fails to connect the body after Dr. Cortner's mutant monster shows up to kill him. At this point it is nothing more than a "Franken" film.

It all seems ridiculous, right? Well, surprise—in 1970, the head of one monkey was transplanted on the body of another monkey, and the monkey lived for a week. That might have been the end of it, but recently a proposal for the first human body-to-head transplantation has been published—the donor a brain dead person, the recipient unclear—but the author suggested a young individual with progressive muscular dystrophy or genetic and metabolic disorders. Whether such a procedure could ever pass an institutional research board is not even a question—it is impossible.

A FINAL WORD

This is just a selection of films but you get the point. Neurofollies gives us the delightful absurdity of comedy and captivating technology of science fiction. Revisiting these films shows that screenwriters have picked up on certain neurologic knowledge, exaggerated it, turned it upside down for entertainment, and placed it into a science fiction category. These filmmakers, I suspect, tried to imagine how the whole fantastical tale could work and how to maximize the fun.

Entertainment, as expected, often wins over reality. Some films are based on books by renowned authors of science fiction and thrillers. Some of these types of films have become cult classics and won Academy Awards. It is amusing and entertaining for its audience, and it is meant to be taken with a grain of salt. However, with the introduction of psychosurgery, brain stimulation for many neurologic disorders, and the use of psychostimulants in stuporous patients, there may be the beginning of some blurring of the lines between reality between current clinical practice and science fiction. But maybe not.

Further Reading

Canavero S. HEAVEN: The head anastomosis venture project outline for the first human head transplantation with spinal linkage (GEMINI). *Surg Neurol Int* 2013;4:S335–42.

Fazel S, Philipson J, Gardiner L, Merritt R, Grann M. Neurological disorders and violence: A systematic review and meta-analysis with a focus on epilepsy and traumatic brain injury. *J Neurol* 2009;256:1591–1602.

Laing O. *The Trip to Echo Spring: On Writers and Drinking.* New York: Picador, 2013.

McDaniel MA, Maier SF, Einstein GO. "Brain-specific" nutrients: A memory cure? *Nutrition* 2003;19:957–75.

Naci L, Monti MM, Cruse D, et al. Brain-computer interfaces for communication with nonresponsive patients. *Ann Neurol* 2012;72:312–23.

Owen AM, Hampshire A, Grahn JA, et al. Putting brain training to the test. *Nature* 2010;465:775–78.

Treiman DM. Epilepsy and violence: Medical and legal issues. *Epilepsia* 1986;27 Suppl 2:S77–104.

White RJ, Wolin LR, Massopust LC, Jr., Taslitz N, Verdura J. Primate cephalic transplantation: Neurogenic separation, vascular association. *Transplant Proc* 1971;3:602–4.

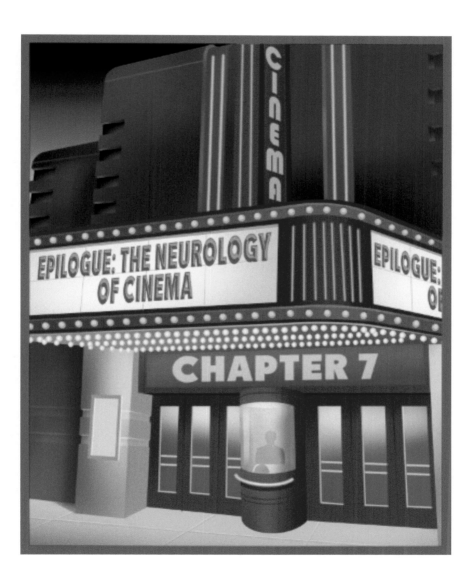

CHAPTER 7

Epilogue

The Neurology of Cinema

No form of art goes beyond ordinary consciousness as film does, straight to our emotions, deep into the twilight room of the soul.

Ingmar Bergman

By the nature of its craft, film impacts emotion and thus memory also. We remember scenes best when emotions are strongly displayed. Emotional narratives filled in with music activate certain parts of the brain. Functional MRI—a technique that records activity and information processing—has shown that watching movies activates the amygdala, a known structure that provides emotional rewards. This happens with funny scenes and in kissing scenes, particularly when combined with a sad or happy soundtrack. Film-induced anxiety or horror movies move the brain activity to the frontal lobe (the anterior cingulate cortex) and thalamus, suggesting increased arousal (a primitive guarding fight response). What movies do to the brain—the light, the dark, the cuts, the shots, the sound—we do not know. What a story line does to a "sick" brain—we do not precisely know either. Why sleep can be troubled after a tense scene remains a mystery. But all these emotions—primal or moral—make cinema dramatically interesting and often unforgettable.

But enough of that, at the end of a film when the closing credits roll, the audience reflects on what just has been shown on the big screen. So, in this final chapter, it is appropriate to further muse on the subtitle of this book, *When Film Meets Neurology*. How do we interpret neurologic portrayal in the movies, and can it be used in teaching? Is the artistic rendering just entertainment and spectacle, or can it have an educational purpose?

There has been some interest in what is called *cinemeducation*. Their case is made by "cinemeducators" that film can be used as a teaching tool. This method relies to a great extent on the cinematic portrayal of medical and social situations, with teachers finding something important to discuss. Most work done in this field—if there is a field—pertains to virtually everything that can potentially be scrutinized when watching film. Leaving out the major illnesses such as cancer, these interpretations have involved a plethora of social- and health-policy issues, couples under emotional duress, strained family behavior, partner violence, aging and frailty, substance abuse, and grieving, as well as the transformative power of loving relationships. These films have been used in college courses on psychology and psychotherapy. Moreover, in counseling sessions, films have also been used to provide relief for patients with a technique known as *cinematherapy*. There is no published systematic study of its benefit or how this method of teaching could effectively fit within a curriculum, and finding and creating video clips may be too complicated for some educators.

Such a broad, all-encompassing approach cannot apply where there is a relatively narrow focus such as in neurocinema. However, thematic films could be helpful in appreciating the major challenges confronting those diagnosed with a neurologic disease. Here are some suggestions on how to most effectively use these films and the resources in this book. But first, how about the actors?

NEUROCINEMA AND ACTORS

Actors often have difficulty portraying the major clinical features of a neurologic disease or symptom. Very few actors have been able to imitate aphasia, and most acted out speech abnormalities are a combination of grunting, clenched teeth, or drunken speech. Walking with a spastic paralyzed leg is done better, but some actors use the cane incorrectly, and at the same side as the paralysis (e.g., *A Simple Life*, Chapter 3). Seizures are difficult to portray for most actors and often involve exaggerated eye quiver, sudden eye deviation upwards, and like "flopping fish out of the water" flailing movements with quick resolution. As we have seen, the representation of a prolonged comatose state remains problematic, with many actors looking well groomed and stunningly fit.

Actors may spend time with patients after acute brain injury, such as stroke patients in rehabilitation centers, and through close observation may acquire some knowledge about their limitations. Such visits may provide insight, but for acute conditions with seriously ill neurologic patients it is not feasible to bring actors into a ward (or intensive care). Screenwriters may contact patient support groups, and I suspect most of the information is coming from these sources.

Little is known about whether neurologists have been consulted for advice, or what advice they have been given. This information may be shown in the closing credits, but often neurologists are not specifically identified, and only a hospital or department is mentioned. Some films are based on patient stories remembered by a neurologist—notably the case histories of Oliver Sacks—but how the screenplays in other films came about remains largely unexplored.

Some actors have been diagnosed with a neurologic disorder. There is no evidence that any of the early symptomatology has impeded their acting, but some actors have used their neurologic disability in a movie (e.g., Rene Kirby with spina bifida is walking on four limbs in the film *Shallow Hal* [2001]).

Michael J. Fox has Parkinson's disease and now also has a Golden Globe-nominated TV show making light of his dyskinetic movements and his Parkinson's disease in general. Michael J. Fox reportedly has said, "I can play anybody, as long as the character has Parkinson's disease." As an example of how actors can contribute significantly to various neurologic causes, Michael J. Fox has started a foundation and has raised millions for research. In 2012, Bob Hoskins, best known for his award-winning role in *Mona Lisa* (1987) and his feature role in *Who Framed Roger Rabbit* (1988), retired from acting because of Parkinson's disease and died in 2014.

Other examples of neurologic disease, but leading to early demise, are David Niven, who developed amyotrophic lateral sclerosis (ALS). Katharine Hepburn was known to have essential tremor, which significantly worsened over the years (note the profound voice tremor and head bobbing in *On Golden Pond* [1981]). The late actor Dudley Moore was markedly impaired by progressive supranuclear palsy, and the late actor and comedian Richard Pryor suffered from multiple sclerosis.

THE BOOK AND WHAT IT MEANS

This book is above all about neurology in film, and after making a determination of how neurology is portrayed in a large number of films, the following observations can be made. Films with neurologic portrayals really started to emerge in the late 1980s, and there has been a steady increase each decade since. This likely is a reflection of the gradual visible appearance of neurology as a specialty, and the stories about neurologic disability that affect us.

All together, after separating the wheat from the chaff, the portrayal captures much of what is important to know about neurology. In about one-third of the films, the portrayal of neurological conditions is excellent, and there is teachable material in many of the films reviewed here. The films are each in their own way interesting. The portrayal of neurologic disease is clearly insufficient in about one-third of the fiction and documentary films reviewed in this book (Figure 7.1). Silly neurology—outside the film genre of horror—can only be found in a handful of films.

In fiction film, there has been an overall improvement in portrayal of neurology over the years. When the number of "mandatory" watching ratings (four reflex hammers) for fiction films is considered separately, there is a fourfold increase since 2000. The increase can be partly explained by the increasing number of films specifically based on a neurologic disease or experience, but you still need the skill of a Daniel Day-Lewis to accurately play the cerebral palsy of Christy Brown, or the caliber of an Al Pacino to personify Jack Kevorkian.

This industry takes notice of accuracy. The entertainment industry, science, and medicine have organized cooperation between two organizations: Hollywood, Health & Society (www.hollywoodhealthandsociety.org) and The Science & Entertainment Exchange (www.scienceandentertainmentexchange.org). These organizations provide scientists and physicians the opportunity to explain biology to the screenwriter. The story line remains mostly untouched, and advisers do not rewrite or edit scripts. Directors may still decide how to present their story, despite being better informed, and whether these organizations are needed or will be helpful in

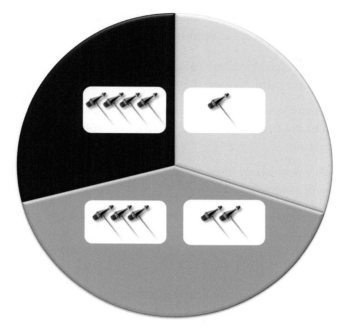

FIGURE 7.1   Ratings of fiction and documentary films discussed in this book (films are listed in the Appendix).

future neurology projects is unknown groups and, I suspect, most of the information is coming from these sources.

HOW TO WATCH AND READ A NEURO FILM

The ultimate goal is to connect the viewing experience with the known reality and to gain more information about neurologic disease. In deciding how to best view and discuss these films, one option is to form a film club. This would allow experts in several subspecialties to evaluate the portrayal and provide context. Films may be watched in small discussion groups, and we at Mayo Clinic have started a combined book and film club alternating neurology in history, neurology in novels, and neurology in the movies.

Documentaries are ideally suited to discuss the challenges of living with (or dying of) a neurologic disease. Important examples are the documentaries on ALS and Alzheimer's disease (Chapter 5). I personally found these documentaries transformative because they show these devastating diseases and their major social consequences in real time.

This book may provide some guidance in discussing some of the films mentioned. Suggestions are as follows (Figure 7.2).

- Discuss the main portrayal and why it is relevant for physicians and neurologists (who may see this every day).

- Discuss an inaccuracy and use it as a teaching advantage. Even a film that does not get it right—and perhaps even more so—could prompt a discussion.

- Discuss a number of films about one topic. By comparing films, patterns will emerge.

- Discuss physician behavior and communication and identify common inappropriately portrayed conversations or lack of compassion. Note offensive or sarcastic remarks of healthcare workers.

- Discuss the major tenets of bioethics in relation to neurologic disease.

- Discuss neurologic disease and human interaction. How do close relatives respond when facing such a crisis? How can we empathize with them?

- Discuss relevant neurologic literature (one or two key papers).

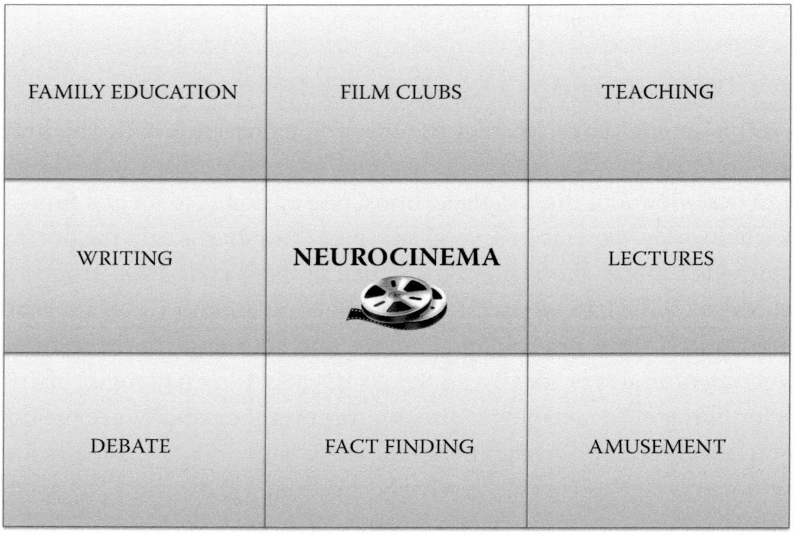

FAMILY EDUCATION	FILM CLUBS	TEACHING
WRITING	NEUROCINEMA	LECTURES
DEBATE	FACT FINDING	AMUSEMENT

FIGURE 7.2   Neurocinema and its possibilities.

CONCLUSION

There is an abundance of great neurofilms. I would be remiss if I did not show the reader my top 10 list of the finest works of neurocinema. For some, these are less common touchstones, but to me, they are "must see."

Something has been achieved when a film incites discussion and further reading. Each of the films discussed in this book demands serious study not only by film scholars, but also by those who see and manage neurologic patients and support their families.

Top 10 Neurocinema:

1. *The Death of Mr. Lazarescu*
2. *Amour*
3. *The Intouchables*
4. *The Diving Bell and the Butterfly*
5. *My Left Foot*
6. *You Don't Know Jack*
7. *Iris*
8. *Memento*
9. *The Crash Reel*
10. *Declaration of War*

Suggested Reading

Alexander M, Pavlov A, Lenahan P. *Cinemeducation: A comprehensive guide to using film in medical education*. Oxford, England: Radcliffe Medical Press, 2005.

Alexander M, Lenahan P, Pavlov A. *Cinemeducation: Using film and other visual media in graduate and medical education*. Vol. 2. Oxford, England: Radcliffe Medical Press, 2012.

Dine Young S. *Psychology at the movies*. Malden, MA: Wiley-Blackwell, 2012.

Glasser B. *Medicinema—Doctors in films*. Abingdon, UK: Oxford, Radcliffe Publishing, 2010.

Hassan A, Wijdicks EFM. Neurology book and film club: The Mayo Clinic experience. *Pract Neurol* 2014,14:68–69.

Pehrs C, Deserno L, Bakels JH, et al. How music alters a kiss: Superior temporal gyrus controls fusiform-amygdalar effective connectivity. *Soc Cogn Affect Neurosci* 2013,Dec 24, published online.

Sawahata Y, Komine K, Morita T, et al. Decoding humor experiences from brain activity of people viewing comedy movies. *PLOS One* 2013,12;e81009.

Solomon G. Reel therapy: How movies inspire you to overcome life's problems. New York: Lebhar-Friedman Books, 2001.

Straube T, Priessler S, Lipka J, et al. Neural representation of anxiety and personality during exposure to anxiety-provoking and neutral scenes from scary movies. *Human Brain Mapping* 2010,31;36–47.

Neurofilmography

This is a full listing of 115 rated films mentioned in this book (not counting the "silly neurology" in Chapter 6) arranged by year of wide release. The major films are presented in boldface. The ratings are defined below. The overall ratings are summarized in a pie graph in Chapter 7.

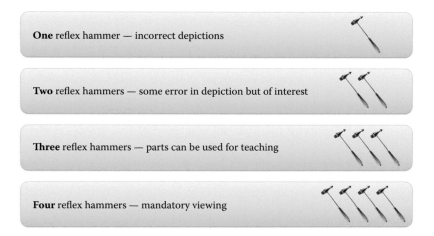

One reflex hammer — incorrect depictions

Two reflex hammers — some error in depiction but of interest

Three reflex hammers — parts can be used for teaching

Four reflex hammers — mandatory viewing

NEUROFILMOGRAPHY (FEATURE FILMS)

Year	Title	Director	Distributor	Rating
1920	*High and Dizzy*	Hal Roach	Pathé Exchange	✎
1939	**Dark Victory**	Edmund Goulding	Warner Brothers	✎
1940	**The Courageous Dr. Christian**	Bernard Vorhaus	Stephens-Lang Productions	✎✎
1945	*Leave Her to Heaven*	John Stahl	Twentieth Century Fox	✎✎✎
1946	**A Matter of Life and Death**	Michael Powell and Emeric Pressburger	Eagle-Lion Films	✎✎✎✎
1946	**Sister Kenny**	Dudley Nichols	RKO Radio Pictures	✎✎✎
1948	*An Act of Murder*	Michael Gorden	Universal Pictures	✎✎
1949	*White Heat*	Raoul Walsh	Warner Brothers	✎
1950	*Crisis*	Richard Brooks	MGM	✎
1950	*The Men*	Fred Zinnemann	United Artists	✎✎✎
1959	*The Five Pennies*	Melville Shavelson	Paramount Pictures	✎
1961	*Viridiana*	Luis Buñuel	Films Sans Frontières	✎
1973	*Turkish Delight*	Paul Verhoeven	VNF	✎✎✎
1975	*The Other Side of the Mountain*	Larry Peerce	Universal Pictures	✎✎✎
1978	*Coming Home*	Hal Ashby	United Artists	✎✎✎
1981	**Whose Life Is It Anyway?**	John Badham	MGM Studios	✎✎✎✎
1987	**Gaby: A True Story**	Luis Mandoki	TriStar Pictures	✎✎
1988	*Rain Man*	Barry Levinson	United Artists	✎✎
1989	*Born on the Fourth of July*	Oliver Stone	Universal Pictures	✎✎
1989	*Drugstore Cowboy*	Gus Van Sant	Avenue Pictures	✎✎✎

NEUROFILMOGRAPHY (FEATURE FILMS) (*Continued*)

Year	Title	Director	Distributor	Rating
1989	*My Left Foot*	Jim Sheridan	Granada Films, Miramax Films	🖉🖉🖉🖉
1989	*Steel Magnolias*	Herbert Ross	TriStar Pictures	🖉🖉🖉
1990	*Awakenings*	Penny Marshall	Columbia Pictures	🖉🖉🖉
1990	*Hard to Kill*	Bruce Malmuth	Warner Brothers	🖉
1990	*Reversal of Fortune*	Barbet Schroeder	Warner Brothers	🖉🖉🖉
1991	*Frankie and Johnny*	Garry Marshall	Paramount Pictures	🖉
1991	*My Own Private Idaho*	Gus Van Sant	Fine Line Features	🖉🖉🖉
1991	*Regarding Henry*	Mike Nichols	Paramount Pictures	🖉
1992	*City of Joy*	Roland Joffé	TriStar Pictures	🖉🖉
1992	*Lorenzo's Oil*	George Miller	Universal Pictures	🖉🖉
1992	*The Waterdance*	Neal Jimenez	Samuel Goldwyn Company	🖉🖉
1994	*Legends of the Fall*	Edward Zwick	TriStar Pictures	🖉
1994	*The Madness of King George*	Nicholas Hytner	Samuel Goldwyn Company	🖉
1995	*Go Now*	Michael Winterbottom	Gramercy Pictures	🖉🖉🖉
1996	*Breaking the Waves*	Lars von Trier	October Films	🖉🖉
1996	*Extreme Measures*	Michael Apted	Columbia Pictures	🖉
1997	*Critical Care*	Sidney Lumet	Mediaworks	🖉🖉🖉🖉
1997	*Firelight*	William Nicholson	Miramax	🖉🖉
1997	*First Do No Harm*	Jim Abrahams	Walt Disney Video	🖉🖉
1997	*Hugo Pool*	Robert Downey, Sr.	Northern Arts Entertainment	🖉

(*Continued*)

NEUROFILMOGRAPHY (FEATURE FILMS) (*Continued*)

Year	Title	Director	Distributor	Rating
1997	*Niagara, Niagara*	Bob Gosse	The Shooting Gallery	🔧
1997	*The Tic Code*	Gary Winick	Lions Gate Entertainment	🔧🔧🔧
1998	*Gods and Monsters*	Bill Condon	Lions Gate Films	🔧🔧
1998	*Hilary and Jackie*	Anand Tucker	Channel 4 Films	🔧🔧
1998	*Pi*	Darren Aronofsky	Artisan Entertainment	🔧🔧
1998	*The Dreamlife of Angels*	Erick Zonca	Sony Pictures	🔧🔧🔧
1998	*The Theory of Flight*	Paul Greengrass	Fine Line Features	🔧
1999	*All About My Mother*	Pedro Almodóvar	Sony Pictures Classics	🔧🔧🔧
1999	*Deuce Bigalow: Male Gigolo*	Mike Mitchell	Buena Vista Pictures	🔧
1999	*Flawless*	Joel Schumacher	MGM	🔧
1999	*Post Concussion*	Daniel Yoon	Blue Water Films	🔧
1999	*Tuesdays with Morrie*	Mick Jackson	Harpo Productions	🔧
2000	*Memento*	Christopher Nolan	Summit Entertainment	🔧🔧🔧
2001	*A Song for Martin*	Bille August	Film i Vast	🔧🔧🔧🔧
2001	*Iris*	Richard Eyre	Miramax Films	🔧🔧🔧🔧
2002	*Door to Door*	Steven Schachter	AOL Time Warner Company	🔧🔧
2002	*Oasis*	Lee Chang-dong	CJ Entertainment	🔧🔧
2002	*Talk to Her*	Pedro Almodóvar	Sony Pictures Classics	🔧
2003	*21 Grams*	Alejandro González Iñárritu	Focus Features	🔧🔧🔧
2003	*Good Bye Lenin!*	Wolfgang Becker	Sony Pictures Classics	🔧

NEUROFILMOGRAPHY (FEATURE FILMS) *(Continued)*

Year	Title	Director	Distributor	Rating
2003	*Matchstick Men*	Ridley Scott	Warner Brothers	🖉🖉
2004	**In Enemy Hands**	Tony Giglio	Lions Gate Entertainment	🖉
2004	*Million Dollar Baby*	Clint Eastwood	Warner Brothers	🖉🖉🖉
2004	*The Machinist*	Brad Anderson	Paramount Vintage	🖉
2004	**The Motorcycle Diaries**	Walter Salles	Focus Features	🖉🖉🖉
2004	*The Notebook*	Nick Cassavetes	New Line Cinema	🖉
2004	**The Sea Inside**	Alejandro Amenábar	Fine Line Features	🖉🖉🖉🖉
2004	*Trauma*	Marc Evans	Warner Brothers	🖉
2005	*The Aura*	Fabián Bielinsky	Buena Vista International IFC Films	🖉🖉🖉
2005	**The Death of Mr. Lazarescu**	Cristi Puiu	Tartan USA	🖉🖉🖉🖉
2006	**Away from Her**	Sarah Polley	Lions Gate Films	🖉🖉🖉🖉
2006	*Memories of Tomorrow*	Yukihiko Tsutsumi	ROAR	🖉🖉
2006	*That Beautiful Somewhere*	Robert Budreau	Loon Films	🖉
2007	**The Diving Bell and the Butterfly**	Julian Schnabel	Pathé Renn Productions, Miramax Films	🖉🖉🖉🖉
2007	**The Lookout**	Scott Frank	Miramax Films	🖉🖉🖉
2007	**The Savages**	Tamara Jenkins	Fox Searchlight Pictures	🖉🖉🖉🖉
2009	**Adam**	Max Mayer	Fox Searchlight Pictures	🖉🖉🖉🖉
2009	**The Cake Eaters**	Mary Stuart Masterson	7-57 Releasing	🖉
2010	**Extraordinary Measures**	Tom Vaughan	CBS Films	🖉

(Continued)

NEUROFILMOGRAPHY (FEATURE FILMS) *(Continued)*

Year	Title	Director	Distributor	Rating
2010	*Love & Other Drugs*	Edward Zwick	20th Century Fox	🔪
2010	**You Don't Know Jack**	Barry Levinson	HBO Films	🔪🔪🔪🔪
2011	**Declaration of War**	Valérie Donzelli	IFC Films	🔪🔪🔪🔪
2011	*Extremely Loud & Incredibly Close*	Stephen Daldry	Warner Brothers	🔪🔪🔪🔪
2011	**Fly Away**	Janet Grillo	New Video Group	🔪🔪🔪🔪
2011	**The Descendants**	Alexander Payne	Fox Searchlight Pictures	🔪🔪🔪🔪
2011	**The Intouchables**	Olivier Nakache	Gaumont Film Company	🔪🔪🔪🔪
2011	**The Music Never Stopped**	Jim Kohlberg	Essential Pictures	🔪🔪🔪🔪
2012	**A Late Quartet**	Yaron Zilberman	Entertainment One	🔪🔪🔪🔪
2012	**A Simple Life**	Ann Hui	Distribution Workshop	🔪🔪🔪
2012	**Amour**	Michael Haneke	Artificial Eye, Sony Pictures Classics	🔪🔪🔪🔪
2012	*Barbara*	Christian Petzold	Schramm Film Koerner & Weber	🔪🔪
2012	*Dormant Beauty*	Marco Bellocchio	Emerging Pictures and Cinema Made in Italy	🔪
2012	**Fred Won't Move Out**	Richard Ledes	Rainwater Films, Ltd.	🔪🔪🔪🔪
2012	**The Sessions**	Ben Lewin	Fox Searchlight Pictures	🔪🔪
2012	**The Vow**	Michael Sucsy	Screen Gems	🔪
2013	**Side Effects**	Steven Soderbergh	Open Roads Films	🔪🔪🔪
2014	**Run & Jump**	Steph Green	Sundance Select	🔪

NEUROFILMOGRAPHY (DOCUMENTARY FILMS)

Year	Title	Director	Distributor	Rating
1998	*A Paralyzing Fear: The Story of Polio in America*	Nina Gilden Seavey	PBS Home Video	✎✎✎✎
2005	*Martha in Lattimore*	Mary Dalton	Wake Forest University	✎✎
2006	*Picturing Aphasia*	Mores McWreath	CreateSpace	✎✎✎
2006	*So Much So Fast*	Steven Ascher and Jeanne Jordan	West City Films	✎✎✎✎
2007	*Coma*	Liz Garbus	Moxie Firecracker Films	✎✎✎
2007	*Living with Lew*	Adam Bardach	Cinetic Media	✎✎✎✎
2010	*Aphasia*	Carl McIntyre	Little Word Films	✎✎
2010	*The Forgetting: A Portrait of Alzheimer's*	Elizabeth Arledge	PBS	✎✎
2012	*Do You Really Want To Know?*	John Zaritsky	Optic Nerve Films	✎✎✎✎
2012	*Extreme Love*	Dan Child	BBC2	✎✎
2012	*You're Looking at Me Like I Live Here and I Don't*	Scott Kirschenbaum	You're Looking at Me, LLC	✎✎✎✎
2013	*After Words*	Vincent Staggas	Flag Day Productions	✎✎✎✎
2013	*I Am Breathing*	Emma Davie and Morag McKinnon	Scottish Documentary Institute	✎✎✎✎
2013	*The Crash Reel*	Lucy Walker	HBO Films	✎✎✎✎
2013	*The Genius of Marian*	Banker White	Capital Film Fund	✎✎✎✎
2013	*When I Walk*	Jason DaSilva	Long Shot Factory	✎✎✎✎
2014	*Alive Inside*	Michael Rossato-Bennett	Bond 360	✎✎✎✎
2014	*Glen Campbell... I'll Be Me*	James Keach	PCH Films	✎✎✎✎

Index